THE MILKY WAY

EXPLORING THE WORLD OF DAIRY

DIPAN KUMAR DAS
SUDIP KUMAR DAS

This book, "The Milky Way: Exploring the World of Dairy," is dedicated to the unsung heroes of the dairy industry—those who toil in the fields, tend to the cows, and transform the humble milk into a rich tapestry of dairy delights. It is a tribute to their hard work, dedication, and unwavering commitment to providing us with nourishing, diverse, and delicious dairy products that enrich our lives in countless ways.

We also dedicate this book to all those who have a deep appreciation for the beauty of dairy, from the artisanal cheesemakers to the passionate bakers, from the dairy scientists pushing the boundaries of innovation to the home cooks experimenting with new recipes. Your love for dairy enriches our culinary experiences and keeps the traditions and culture of dairy alive.

Last but not least, we dedicate this book to every reader, young and old, who embarks on this journey through "The Milky Way." Your curiosity and willingness to explore the world of dairy, its history, science, and cultural significance, are the driving force behind the continued appreciation and preservation of this remarkable industry.

May this book inspire you to celebrate and savor the world of dairy in all its forms, from the cow to your glass and beyond.

Foreword

In a world teeming with culinary delights and a treasure trove of flavors, dairy products stand out as a cornerstone of gastronomy. From the nourishing glass of milk to the exquisite bite of a perfectly aged cheese, dairy has woven its way into the fabric of our diets and cultures. The story of dairy is a tale of agriculture, science, and artistry that has unfolded over millennia, and it continues to evolve in our modern world.

As we embark on a journey through "The Milky Way: Exploring the World of Dairy," we invite you to savor the richness and complexity of this remarkable industry. Whether you are a passionate foodie, a dairy aficionado, or simply curious about the story behind your favorite dairy products, this book will guide you through the pastures, farms, and kitchens that have shaped the world of dairy.

We will travel back in time to explore the origins of dairy farming, uncover the practices and innovations that have transformed milk into an array of dairy delights, and celebrate the health benefits and cultural significance of dairy. Along the way, we will encounter the diverse and dynamic universe of dairy products, from the velvety creams to the tangy yogurts, from the flavorful cheeses to the timeless classics like butter and milk.

"The Milky Way" is a celebration of the people, traditions, and innovations that have propelled the dairy industry forward. It is a testament to the enduring significance of dairy in our lives, from nurturing our bodies with essential nutrients to tantalizing our taste buds with a world of flavors. It is a journey that will take you from the origins of dairy farming to the innovations of the future.

So, as we set forth on this odyssey through the Milky Way, we invite you to savor every page, to explore the diverse and rich world of dairy, and to deepen your appreciation for the dairy products that enrich our lives and our culinary traditions.

Bon appétit, and may your exploration of "The Milky Way" be as enriching and delightful as the dairy it celebrates.

Preface

In the realm of culinary delights, few things are as rich and diverse as dairy products. From a simple glass of milk to the intricate craftsmanship of a well-aged cheese, the world of dairy is a universe of flavors, textures, and traditions waiting to be explored. The journey through "The Milky Way: Exploring the World of Dairy" is an invitation to embark on a voyage that uncovers the beauty, history, and significance of this extraordinary industry.

Dairy is not just about what we find in the supermarket; it's about the pastures and the cows, the hands that milk them, the artisans who transform the milk into cheese, the scientists who study its properties, and the chefs who create culinary masterpieces with it. It's a story that weaves together the traditions of ancient cultures, the innovations of modern science, and the ever-evolving culinary arts.

This book is a celebration of all things dairy, from the farm to the table, from the science to the culture. It's an exploration of the connections between what we consume and where it comes from, between the flavors we savor and the history that brought them to our plates. It's a journey that will reveal the rich tapestry of dairy in all its forms, from the familiar to the exotic, from the comforting to the daring.

As you embark on this expedition through the Milky Way, we invite you to savor every page, to discover the wonders of the dairy world, and to deepen your appreciation for the dairy products that grace our meals and enrich our lives. Whether you're a seasoned cheese connoisseur, a curious home cook, or simply someone who enjoys a scoop of ice cream on a sunny day, there's something in this journey for you.

So, let us set forth on this exploration of "The Milky Way." May it be as nourishing, as delightful, and as enlightening as the dairy it celebrates.

Prologue

In a world filled with an abundance of flavors, textures, and culinary traditions, the story of dairy unfolds as a remarkable odyssey of nourishment, culture, and craftsmanship. This book, "The Milky Way: Exploring the World of Dairy," is an invitation to embark on a journey through the rich and diverse universe of dairy products.

The story of dairy is a story of humanity's enduring relationship with nature, where milk from cows, goats, and sheep has nourished generations and left its mark on cultures across the globe. It is a story of innovation, where the art of cheesemaking, the science of fermentation, and the mastery of butter-churning have been honed to perfection.

Dairy is a story of nutrition, where the wholesome glass of milk offers essential nutrients for growth and vitality. It is a story of culture, where each cheese, each yogurt, and each butter carries the legacy of the people and places that crafted them. It is a story of health, where dairy products contribute to bone strength, cardiovascular wellness, and overall well-being.

The journey through "The Milky Way" will take us from the pastoral landscapes where cows graze and sheep roam, to the bustling dairy farms where milking machines hum, and to the artisanal creameries where cheese wheels age to perfection. We will uncover the history, science, and cultural significance of dairy, exploring the links between what we consume and the world that produces it.

As we set forth on this odyssey through the Milky Way, we invite you to savor every page, to explore the diverse and rich world of dairy, and to deepen your appreciation for the dairy products that grace our tables. Whether you are a passionate foodie, a culinary enthusiast, or simply someone who enjoys the comforting taste of a scoop of ice cream, there is something in this journey for you.

So, let us begin this exploration of "The Milky Way." May it be as enriching, as enlightening, and as delightful as the dairy it celebrates.

Foreword

Preface

Prologue

CHAPTER ONE

From Pasture to Parlor

In the opening chapter of "The Milky Way: Exploring the World of Dairy," we embark on a journey that unveils the intricate path dairy products take from the lush pastures to our homes. This chapter serves as a foundational exploration of the dairy industry, shedding light on the stages and processes that bring dairy to our tables.

The chapter commences with an introduction to the central role that dairy plays in human nutrition and cultural traditions worldwide. It sets the stage for the captivating journey through the dairy world, beginning with the pastoral scenes of dairy farms and the cows that provide the primary source of milk.

Readers are introduced to the heart of dairy farming, where cows graze on open pastures, providing fresh, raw milk. The process of milking, which is a skilled and often daily ritual, is explained, offering insight into the connection between dairy farmers and their herds.

From there, the story moves to the transportation of the raw milk to processing facilities. Readers will gain an understanding of the meticulous standards and protocols in place to ensure the safety and quality of the milk before it reaches the processing plants.

The chapter will also touch on the critical issue of dairy farm sustainability, discussing environmentally friendly practices and ethical considerations in the industry. Modern advancements, such as automated milking systems and sustainable agriculture techniques, will be highlighted.

As the chapter draws to a close, the focus shifts to the processing and packaging of milk and its various by-products, which are then shipped to consumers' homes or local stores. This section will emphasize the importance of freshness and quality control in the dairy supply chain.

"From Pasture to Parlor" sets the stage for the in-depth exploration of the dairy world that follows in subsequent chapters, painting a vivid picture of the journey that dairy takes from the serene pastures where it begins to the cozy parlor where it becomes a staple in our daily lives.

The chapter also delves into the human aspect of dairy farming. It explores the dedication and hard work of dairy farmers, whose livelihoods are intertwined with their herds and the land they steward. The bonds formed between farmers and their animals are illuminated, providing readers with a deeper appreciation of the individuals behind the milk production process.

Readers will gain insights into the challenges faced by dairy farmers, including the ever-evolving agricultural landscape, market fluctuations, and the importance of animal welfare. These challenges emphasize the resilience and adaptability of the dairy industry throughout its history.

Throughout "From Pasture to Parlor," readers are encouraged to reflect on the connections between the origins of dairy and its significance in their own lives. The chapter aims to foster an appreciation for the dedication and hard work that goes into providing high-quality dairy products, as well as the importance of sustainable practices that safeguard the environment for future generations.

In this first chapter, readers are not only introduced to the journey of dairy but are also prompted to contemplate the pivotal role that dairy plays in our lives and the communities that depend on it. The book unfolds to explore the rich tapestry of the dairy world, offering readers a comprehensive understanding of the complexities and beauty of the dairy industry.

As readers progress through the chapter, they'll gain a broader perspective on the global significance of dairy, touching upon the diverse cultural traditions and culinary uses of dairy products. The chapter will highlight how dairy transcends geographical boundaries, enriching the diets and cultures of people around the world.

Furthermore, the chapter will explore the role of technology and innovation in modern dairy farming and processing. It will showcase the ways in which cutting-edge technologies have enhanced efficiency, product quality, and sustainability in the dairy industry. This includes automated milking systems, advanced quality control measures, and sustainable farming practices.

The environmental impact of dairy production will also be discussed. Readers will discover how dairy farmers and producers are increasingly implementing eco-friendly practices, such as reducing greenhouse gas emissions and minimizing waste, to address environmental concerns.

Finally, the chapter will address the growing interest in organic and locally-sourced dairy products, reflecting the changing consumer preferences for more sustainable and ethically produced goods. This growing trend highlights the importance of transparency and traceability in the dairy supply chain.

"From Pasture to Parlor" will not only serve as an introduction to the world of dairy but also as a gateway to the deeper exploration of the topics covered in subsequent chapters. Readers will be left with a profound appreciation for the journey that milk takes from the serene pastures to their own parlor, fostering a greater understanding of the dairy industry and its global significance.

The chapter will also emphasize the importance of regulatory standards and quality control in the dairy industry. Readers will gain an understanding of the stringent measures in place to ensure that dairy products meet the highest standards of safety and quality before they reach consumers' homes. This includes topics like pasteurization, homogenization, and rigorous testing.

One of the key takeaways from this chapter is the integral role of milk in human history. The journey of milk from pasture to parlor is not only a modern marvel but a tradition that spans thousands of years. Readers will be invited to explore the historical roots of dairy farming, from its origins in ancient civilizations to its transformation into a global industry.

Additionally, the chapter will feature anecdotes and stories from dairy farmers, highlighting their commitment to their craft, the challenges they face, and the rewards they reap. These personal accounts will add a human element to the story of dairy, making it relatable and engaging for readers.

Finally, "From Pasture to Parlor" will lay the groundwork for the subsequent chapters, which will delve deeper into the various aspects of dairy production, processing, nutrition, and its impact on health, culture, and the environment. It will encourage readers to approach the rest of the book with a renewed appreciation for the journey of dairy products from the serene pastures where it all begins to the comforting parlor where it becomes a beloved part of our daily lives.

Introduction: The Journey of Milk from Cow to Glass

In the heart of the dairy industry lies a remarkable and intricate journey, one that transforms a humble liquid into a daily staple cherished by people around the world. This journey, the passage of milk from the cow to your glass, is a testament to the dedication of dairy farmers, the marvels of modern technology, and the enduring relationship between humans and bovines. In this book, "The Milky Way: Exploring the World of Dairy," we embark on a voyage that unveils the enchanting world of dairy, beginning with this introduction, where we trace the fascinating odyssey of milk.

The dairy industry is not just about bottles on supermarket shelves; it's a tapestry of history, tradition, science, and innovation. As we begin our journey, let's envision a sprawling pasture, where contented cows graze under the open sky, each day contributing the primary source of this white elixir.

Our first stop on this journey is the farm, where we witness the harmonious relationship between dairy farmers and their cows. The milking process is not merely a chore but an art form, where experienced hands deftly coax the milk from the udders, forging a connection that has existed for centuries.

From the farm, we move on to the processing facilities. Here, the milk undergoes a transformation, with careful pasteurization and quality control measures to ensure that the milk you receive is safe and pure. It is at these facilities that the liquid is molded into an array of dairy products, from creamy cheeses to rich butter and velvety yogurts.

The journey then leads us to the grocery store, where you, the consumer, make the final selection of your preferred dairy products. In the comfort of your home, these products become a part of your daily life, offering nutrition, flavor, and versatility.

Throughout this book, we will delve deeper into each stage of this incredible journey, exploring the history of dairy farming, the various dairy cow breeds, the art of cheese-making, the cultural significance of dairy in our world, and the innovations that drive the industry forward. We'll also discuss the nutritional value of milk and its role in human health.

Our journey will not only take us through the physical transformation of milk but also through the cultural and scientific aspects that shape the dairy industry. So, fasten your seatbelt and prepare to embark on "The Milky Way," where we will uncover the rich and diverse world of dairy, from the tranquil pastures to the comfort of your parlor.

The journey of milk from cow to glass is not just a physical process; it's a story of tradition, innovation, and the profound connection between humans, animals, and the land. It's a story of how an ancient source of nourishment has evolved into a dynamic and ever-changing industry that touches the lives of billions.

As we delve deeper into the chapters that follow, we'll learn about the diverse breeds of dairy cows, each with its unique qualities and contributions. We'll explore the world of cheese, from the pungent blues to the creamy bries, and how these creations have left an indelible mark on culinary traditions across the globe. Butter, cream, yogurt, and other dairy delights will each take their turn in the spotlight, revealing their culinary versatility and cultural significance.

We will also discuss the intersection of dairy and human health, addressing the benefits and controversies surrounding dairy consumption, as well as providing insights into alternatives for those with dietary restrictions.

This journey will not only take us from cow to glass but also into the wider world. We'll investigate the surprising uses of dairy in various non-food industries, from cosmetics to textiles, showcasing the versatility of milk and its by-products.

Moreover, the future of dairy farming and production will be a central theme. We will examine the sustainability efforts and technological innovations that are shaping the industry's path toward a more environmentally friendly and efficient future.

Through this exploration, we hope to foster a deep appreciation for the dairy industry, from the dedication of farmers and the craftsmanship of artisans to the nourishing and delightful products that find their way to our tables.

So, with this introduction as our starting point, let's embark on an enlightening and enriching journey through the Milky Way, where we will explore the multifaceted world of dairy, from its roots in the pasture to its place in our parlor, and discover the countless ways it enriches our lives.

CHAPTER TWO

The History of Dairy Farming

Dairy farming is more than just a modern agricultural practice; it is a tradition that spans thousands of years, deeply woven into the fabric of human history. In this chapter, we will take a journey through time, tracing the roots of dairy farming from its earliest origins to the sophisticated industry we know today.

The Dawn of Dairy Farming

To truly appreciate dairy farming, we must venture back to its beginnings. We'll explore how ancient civilizations, such as the Sumerians and Egyptians, first discovered the value of milk from domesticated animals. The chapter will reveal how these early dairy pioneers not only depended on milk for sustenance but also recognized its potential to be transformed into products like cheese and butter.

The dawn of dairy farming can be traced back thousands of years to the Neolithic period, when humans transitioned from a nomadic, hunter-gatherer lifestyle to a more settled, agrarian one. During this time, people began domesticating animals for various purposes, including milk production. Here's a brief overview of the history of dairy farming:

Domestication of Livestock: Around 10,000 years ago, in regions like the Fertile Crescent (modern-day Iraq and Iran), people began domesticating animals such as goats, sheep, and cattle. These animals were kept not only for their meat and hides but also for their milk.

Early Dairy Practices: Initially, early dairy farmers may have been semi-nomadic, following their herds and practicing seasonal transhumance. They would have recognized the nutritional value of milk and learned to process it into products like cheese and yogurt to extend its shelf life.

Development of Agriculture: As agriculture developed, dairy farming became more centralized. People began cultivating crops to feed their livestock, and the practice of milking animals became more sophisticated.

Ancient Civilizations: Various ancient civilizations, including the Egyptians, Greeks, and Romans, incorporated dairy farming into their way of life. They developed cheese-making techniques, created dairy products like butter, and recognized the importance of milk in their diets.

Middle Ages: In Europe, during the Middle Ages, monasteries played a significant role in advancing dairy farming. Monks refined cheese-making techniques and developed new varieties of cheese.

The Dairy Revolution: The Dairy Revolution, which took place in the 18th and 19th centuries, saw significant advancements in dairy farming. Innovations like the milking machine, pasteurization, and refrigeration improved milk quality and storage. This period also witnessed the development of large-scale commercial dairy farms.

Modern Dairy Farming: Today, dairy farming is a vital component of agriculture in many countries. It has become highly industrialized, with large-scale commercial operations producing milk, cheese, butter, and various other dairy products. Milk is processed and distributed to consumers worldwide.

Dairy farming has come a long way since its early beginnings, and it continues to evolve with advancements in technology and changing consumer preferences. Sustainability and animal welfare have become important considerations in modern dairy farming practices, with a focus on ethical treatment of animals and minimizing environmental impact.

From Milking Pails to Milking Machines

The history of dairy farming is a tale of continual innovation. We will discuss the evolution of milking methods, from the humble pail and stool to the invention of the milking machine, which revolutionized the industry. These developments not only increased efficiency but also improved the welfare of dairy animals.

The transition from milking pails to milking machines represents a significant technological advancement in dairy farming. Milking machines have revolutionized the dairy industry, making the milking process more efficient, hygienic, and less labor-intensive. Here's an overview of this transition:

Early Milking Methods: In the early days of dairy farming, milking was done by hand using milking pails or buckets. Farmers or farmworkers would manually milk the cows, goats, or other dairy animals. This process was time-consuming, physically demanding, and often led to variations in milk quality and yield.

The Invention of Milking Machines: The concept of milking machines dates back to the late 18th century, but it wasn't until the 19th and early 20th centuries that functional milking machines were developed. Several inventors contributed to the development of these machines, including Anna Baldwin and Gustaf de Laval.

Types of Milking Machines: There are two main types of milking machines: bucket milking machines and pipeline milking machines.

Bucket Milking Machines: These early milking machines featured a system of cups and pulsators connected to a milk bucket. The operator would attach the cups to the cow's udder, and the machine would automatically milk the cow. The milk would be collected in a bucket, making it easier to handle and transport.

Pipeline Milking Machines: Pipeline milking machines, also known as continuous-flow milking machines, replaced the bucket with a network of pipes and a centralized milk collection system. Milk is directly transported from the udder through a vacuum system and pipelines to a storage tank, bypassing the need for manual collection in buckets.

Advantages of Milking Machines:

Efficiency: Milking machines are faster than manual milking, allowing dairy farmers to milk more cows in less time.

Hygiene: Milking machines are designed to maintain higher levels of cleanliness and reduce the risk of contamination compared to traditional pails.

Consistency: Milking machines provide more consistent milking pressure and can detect irregularities in milk production, helping identify health issues in cows.

Labor Savings: The use of milking machines reduces the physical labor required for milking, which can be particularly beneficial for larger dairy operations.

Modern Milking Machines: Over time, milking machines have continued to evolve with technological advancements. Today's milking machines are highly automated and equipped with sensors, monitoring systems, and data analysis tools to optimize milking efficiency and animal health.

The adoption of milking machines has transformed dairy farming, making it a more efficient and productive industry. These machines have significantly increased milk production capacity and quality while reducing the physical strain on dairy farmers. However, it's important to note that proper training and maintenance are crucial to ensure the well-being of the animals and the quality of the milk.

The Role of Dairy in Different Cultures

Dairy farming has a rich tapestry of cultural significance. We will explore how different cultures around the world have integrated dairy into their traditions and cuisine. From the creamy ghee of India to the tangy yogurt of the Middle East, dairy has played a vital role in global culinary traditions.

Dairy plays a significant role in various cultures around the world, although the types of dairy products consumed, their cultural significance, and their preparation methods can vary widely. Here's a look at the role of dairy in different cultures:

Western Cultures (Europe and North America):

Milk and Cheese: In Western cultures, dairy products such as milk and cheese are staples. They are commonly consumed in various forms, from fresh milk to a wide variety of cheese types like cheddar, mozzarella, and brie.

Butter: Butter is used for cooking, baking, and as a condiment.

Yogurt: Yogurt is often consumed as a snack or breakfast item, and it's a common ingredient in dips and dressings.

Cream: Heavy cream and sour cream are used in cooking and as condiments.

Ice Cream: Ice cream is a popular dessert in Western countries.

Mediterranean and Middle Eastern Cultures:

Cheese: Cheese, especially feta, halloumi, and labneh, is commonly used in Mediterranean and Middle Eastern cuisine.

Yogurt: Yogurt is used in both sweet and savory dishes, such as tzatziki, and is often served with honey and fruit as a dessert.

Butter and Ghee: Butter is used in cooking, while ghee (clarified butter) is a key ingredient in many Indian and Middle Eastern dishes.

Milk-Based Desserts: Desserts like baklava and rice pudding often feature milk or yogurt.

Indian Culture:

Milk: Milk is a crucial ingredient in Indian cuisine and is used in various traditional dishes, such as paneer (Indian cheese), ghee, and various sweets.

Yogurt: Yogurt, known as dahi, is widely used in Indian cooking and is used to make popular dishes like raita and lassi.

Paneer: A fresh cheese made from milk, paneer is a key ingredient in many Indian vegetarian dishes.

African Cultures:

Milk: In some African cultures, milk, often from cows, goats, or camels, is consumed directly or used to make products like sour milk or fermented milk.

Cheese: Varieties of cheese, such as jben in North Africa, are enjoyed in different parts of the continent.

Asian Cultures:

Milk: In some Asian countries like Mongolia and parts of India, milk from animals like yaks and water buffaloes is a dietary staple.

Paneer and Ghee: Paneer is popular in South Asian cuisine, while ghee is widely used for cooking in Indian and Southeast Asian dishes.

Nordic and Scandinavian Cultures:

Dairy Products: Dairy plays a significant role in Nordic cuisine. Products like skyr (a type of yogurt), cheese, and various milk-based dishes are traditional in these regions.

Agricultural and Pastoral Societies:

In many pastoral societies, dairy products are a primary food source. Nomadic cultures often rely on milk, cheese, and other dairy products from their livestock.

Cultural Celebrations: In numerous cultures, dairy-based foods are central to celebrations and rituals. For example, cheese is a vital part of Swiss fondue, and yogurt and butter are featured in Indian wedding feasts.

It's important to note that cultural practices and dietary preferences vary widely, and not all individuals within a culture may consume dairy products due to dietary restrictions, allergies, or personal choices. Nevertheless, dairy products continue to hold cultural significance and provide important nutritional value in many parts of the world.

The Transition to Industrialization

With the onset of the Industrial Revolution, dairy farming underwent a significant transformation. The chapter will delve into how advancements in transportation, refrigeration, and processing revolutionized the dairy industry, leading to the widespread availability of dairy products.

The transition to industrialization was a profound and transformative period in human history. It marked a shift from agrarian and handicraft-based economies to industrial and mechanized systems. This transition had far-reaching impacts on society, the economy, and technology. Here's an overview of this transition:

Agricultural Revolution: Before industrialization, societies were primarily agrarian, with most people engaged in farming and producing food. The agricultural revolution in the 18th century saw advancements in farming techniques, such as crop rotation and selective breeding of livestock, leading to increased agricultural productivity.

Invention of Machinery: One of the pivotal moments in industrialization was the development of new machinery. The mechanization of various industries, beginning with textiles, played a critical role. Inventions like the spinning jenny and the power loom revolutionized the textile industry, making it more efficient and leading to the growth of factories.

Factory System: The factory system emerged as a core feature of industrialization. Large factories and mills centralized production, allowing for economies of scale and the utilization of machinery to increase output. This resulted in the migration of people from rural areas to cities in search of work.

Technological Advances: Alongside the textile industry, the industrial revolution saw significant technological advancements in transportation (e.g., the steam engine and locomotives) and iron and steel production. These innovations powered the growth of various industries.

Urbanization: As industrialization progressed, urbanization followed. Cities grew rapidly as people moved to urban areas in search of employment in the factories and mills. This shift led to the growth of urban centers and the development of infrastructure like roads, bridges, and housing.

Social Changes: Industrialization brought about significant social changes. The traditional family-based economic structure gave way to a more individualistic and wage-based system. Labor unions formed to advocate for workers' rights, as labor conditions were often harsh.

Economic Transformation: Industrialization transformed economies from subsistence-based to market-based. It led to the development of capitalism, with entrepreneurs and business owners investing in and profiting from industrial enterprises.

Impact on Agriculture: As more people moved to cities, there was a decrease in the agricultural workforce. However, mechanization and technological advancements in agriculture also improved productivity on farms.

Education and Science: The demand for a more skilled and literate workforce led to advancements in education. Scientific discoveries and inventions, such as electricity and the telegraph, further accelerated the industrialization process.

Global Impact: Industrialization had global ramifications, as industrialized nations sought raw materials and new markets for their products. It contributed to the growth of imperialism and colonialism, where European powers established colonies to secure resources.

Environmental Consequences: Industrialization had both positive and negative environmental impacts. It led to increased pollution, deforestation, and resource extraction but also enabled advancements in sanitation and public health.

Long-Term Effects: Industrialization continues to shape the modern world, as it laid the foundation for technological progress, economic development, and the rise of the modern global economy.

It's important to note that the industrialization process was not uniform across all countries and regions, and its effects were often accompanied by significant social and political challenges, including labor unrest and the struggle for workers' rights. However, it ultimately reshaped the world and set the stage for the modern era.

Challenges and Controversies

The history of dairy farming is not without its challenges and controversies. We will discuss the economic and ethical issues that have arisen over the years, including concerns about animal welfare, environmental impact, and the consolidation of dairy production.

The transition to industrialization brought about significant challenges and controversies, many of which continue to shape societal debates and policies. Some of the key challenges and controversies associated with industrialization include:

Labor Exploitation: The rapid growth of factories and urbanization often led to harsh working conditions, long hours, and low wages for laborers, including women and children. Labor exploitation sparked the labor movement, trade unions, and demands for workers‘ rights and safer working conditions.

Child Labor: The use of child labor in factories and mines was a major controversy. Child labor was widespread, and reform movements emerged to address this issue, ultimately leading to child labor laws and compulsory education.

Environmental Degradation: Industrialization brought about pollution, deforestation, and resource depletion. The contamination of air and water and the loss of natural habitats raised concerns about environmental sustainability and the long-term consequences of industrialization.

Urbanization Challenges: Rapid urbanization resulted in overcrowded and unsanitary living conditions, leading to public health crises. The lack of infrastructure, such as clean water and sanitation, posed significant challenges in cities.

Social Inequality: Industrialization often exacerbated social inequality, with a small elite class benefiting from economic growth while many workers lived in poverty. Social reforms and movements for equality emerged in response.

Technological Displacement: The mechanization of industries led to job displacement for some workers, particularly in traditional crafts and manual labor. This displacement raised concerns about economic inequality and the need for retraining and education.

Cultural Disruption: The shift from agrarian, community-based societies to urban, industrialized ones resulted in significant cultural disruptions.

Traditional values, social structures, and family dynamics changed, leading to debates about cultural preservation and adaptation.

Impact on Agriculture: Industrialization led to changes in agriculture, with increased mechanization and consolidation of farms. This transformation had mixed effects, including increased food production but also the displacement of rural populations.

Global Consequences: The pursuit of resources and markets by industrialized nations contributed to imperialism and colonialism. This expansion had far-reaching consequences, including cultural clashes and the exploitation of colonized peoples.

Technology and Ethical Dilemmas: The development of new technologies during industrialization, such as the steam engine and electricity, raised ethical questions about their use and potential for harm, as well as the responsibility of scientists and inventors.

Consumerism and Materialism: Industrialization and the growth of consumer culture raised concerns about materialism, overconsumption, and the impact on human values and social priorities.

Political and Ideological Conflicts: Industrialization gave rise to political ideologies such as Marxism and capitalism, leading to ideological conflicts and debates about the role of government in regulating the economy and addressing social issues.

Public Health and Safety: The influx of people into crowded cities created public health challenges, including disease outbreaks. Advances in public health and sanitation were essential to address these issues.

Ethical Treatment of Animals: As industrialization transformed agriculture, concerns about the ethical treatment of animals in factory farming and the impact on animal welfare became increasingly prominent.

These challenges and controversies associated with industrialization have shaped the development of modern societies, led to social and political reforms, and continue to be subjects of debate and reform efforts. Balancing economic development with social and environmental considerations remains a central challenge in the ongoing process of industrialization.

The Resilience of Dairy Farming

Despite the challenges, dairy farming has persevered and adapted. We will highlight the resilience of dairy farmers and the industry as a whole, showcasing how it has continued to provide essential nourishment to people around the world.

Dairy farming has demonstrated remarkable resilience over the years, adapting to changing economic, technological, and environmental conditions. This resilience can be attributed to several factors:

Diverse Dairy Products: Dairy farming produces a wide range of products, including milk, cheese, butter, yogurt, and more. This diversity allows dairy farmers to adapt to shifting consumer preferences and market demands. For example, the popularity of Greek yogurt in recent years has created new opportunities for dairy producers.

Technological Advancements: Dairy farming has benefited from technological innovations, such as automated milking machines, improved herd management systems, and genetic selection tools. These advancements have increased productivity and efficiency, making dairy farming more resilient in the face of labor shortages and other challenges.

Sustainable Practices: Many dairy farms have embraced sustainable and environmentally friendly practices. They focus on reducing their carbon footprint, managing waste, and conserving resources. Sustainable practices not only benefit the environment but also help dairy farms remain economically viable in a world increasingly concerned about climate change.

Diversification: Some dairy farms have diversified their operations to include agritourism, on-farm sales of dairy products, or complementary agricultural activities. This diversification spreads risk and helps farms remain financially stable.

Research and Education: The dairy industry invests in research and education to improve animal welfare, milk quality, and farm management practices. Continuous learning and adaptation to new knowledge help dairy farmers address emerging challenges.

Quality Assurance: Dairy farms often participate in quality assurance programs and certifications, ensuring that their products meet high standards of safety and quality. These programs build consumer trust and allow farms to maintain market access.

Government Support: In many countries, government support programs provide financial assistance, education, and resources to dairy farmers during challenging times. These programs help stabilize the industry during economic downturns or crises.

Global Markets: The dairy industry is part of the global food supply chain. Dairy products are traded internationally, and this global reach can provide opportunities for dairy farmers to access larger markets and diversify income sources.

Consumer Demand for Dairy Products: Despite changing dietary trends and concerns about lactose intolerance, there is a continued and often growing demand for dairy products. This demand can provide a stable market for dairy farmers.

Adaptation to Health Trends: Dairy farmers have adapted to changing health trends by offering lactose-free and plant-based dairy alternatives. This flexibility ensures that dairy farming can cater to various dietary preferences.

Resilience in the Face of Challenges: Dairy farming has faced numerous challenges, including price fluctuations, disease outbreaks, and changing regulations. The industry's ability to persevere and adapt to these challenges showcases its resilience.

Community Support: Many dairy farms are deeply ingrained in their local communities. This sense of community support can be a valuable resource in times of need, providing assistance, advice, and a network for sharing information.

The resilience of dairy farming reflects the industry's ability to evolve and adapt to changing circumstances while continuing to provide essential dairy products to consumers. By embracing innovation, sustainability, and best practices, dairy farmers have maintained their position as important contributors to the global food supply.

Scientific Advancements and Understanding

Scientific advancements and understanding have played a crucial role in the dairy industry, leading to improved production practices, the development of new dairy products, and a better understanding of the nutritional and health aspects of dairy consumption. Here are some key areas in which science has made significant contributions to the dairy sector:

Animal Genetics and Breeding: Advances in genetics and genomics have enabled dairy farmers to selectively breed animals for higher milk production, disease resistance, and other desirable traits. This has led to the development of dairy breeds optimized for various purposes, such as high-yield Holsteins or dual-purpose Jerseys.

Nutritional Science: Scientific research has deepened our understanding of the nutritional composition of dairy products. This knowledge has not only contributed to improved animal nutrition but also provided consumers with a better understanding of the health benefits of dairy consumption. For instance, dairy products are rich sources of essential nutrients like calcium, vitamin D, and high-quality protein.

Quality Control and Safety: Dairy scientists have developed advanced quality control measures to ensure the safety and quality of dairy products. This includes testing for pathogens, monitoring milk composition, and developing protocols for pasteurization and sterilization to extend shelf life.

Milk Processing Technology: Innovations in milk processing technology have enabled the development of various dairy products, such as yogurt, cheese, and butter. These products undergo precise and controlled processes to achieve specific textures and flavors.

Milk Production Efficiency: Research in dairy nutrition, animal health, and management practices has increased the efficiency of milk production. Farmers can optimize feed formulations, improve animal health, and manage herd genetics to maximize milk yield while minimizing resource use.

Sustainable Practices: Scientific advancements have also contributed to the adoption of more sustainable dairy farming practices. Researchers have developed methods to reduce environmental impacts, such as optimizing manure management, energy efficiency, and waste reduction.

Biotechnology: Biotechnology, including the use of recombinant bovine somatotropin (rBST), has been applied to increase milk production per cow. This has been a subject of controversy due to concerns about animal welfare and human health, but it illustrates the influence of scientific advancements on dairy farming.

Microbiology and Starter Cultures: In cheese and yogurt production, understanding the microbiology of fermentation and the use of specific starter cultures have resulted in consistent product quality and a wide range of cheese and yogurt varieties.

Lactose Intolerance and Dairy Alternatives: Research into lactose intolerance has led to a better understanding of this condition and the development of lactose-free dairy products. It has also contributed to the rise of dairy alternatives, such as almond milk and soy milk, and the science behind their production.

Consumer Preferences and Trends: Advances in market research and consumer science have helped dairy producers tailor their products to meet consumer preferences and emerging dietary trends, such as low-fat, organic, or functional dairy products.

Health and Wellness Benefits: Ongoing research into the potential health benefits of dairy consumption, including its role in bone health, muscle growth, and weight management, has provided a scientific foundation for promoting dairy as part of a balanced diet.

Dairy Farming and World Trade

The history of dairy farming is intertwined with the history of trade and globalization. We will discuss how the demand for dairy products led to the establishment of dairy trade networks, contributing to the spread of dairy farming practices and the exchange of knowledge across borders.

The history of dairy farming and world trade are indeed closely intertwined. The demand for dairy products has been a driving force behind trade networks, globalization, and the spread of dairy farming practices and knowledge. Here are key points that illustrate this connection:

Early Dairy Trade: Dairy products like cheese and butter have been traded across regions for centuries. In ancient times, the Roman Empire was known for its cheese production, and it exported cheese to various parts of Europe. Similarly, in Asia, the trading of dairy products was common along the Silk Road and other trade routes.

European Expansion: As European powers expanded their colonial empires, dairy farming and dairy products were introduced to new parts of the world. European settlers often brought dairy cattle and farming techniques with them, contributing to the spread of dairy farming practices in regions such as North and South America, Africa, and Asia.

Global Dairy Trade: The global dairy trade has become a significant component of international commerce. Countries with abundant dairy resources, such as New Zealand and the United States, export dairy products like milk powder, cheese, and butter to countries with high demand but limited local production.

International Dairy Organizations: Organizations like the International Dairy Federation (IDF) and the Global Dairy Platform (GDP) play a vital role in promoting international cooperation, setting quality standards, and facilitating information exchange among dairy-producing nations. They work to harmonize dairy practices and foster collaboration in research and development.

Technology Transfer: The globalization of dairy farming has led to the exchange of knowledge and technology. For example, advanced milking machines, animal genetics, and dairy processing equipment developed in one country can quickly find their way into dairy operations around the world. This technology transfer has contributed to increased productivity and efficiency.

Cultural Exchange: The trade of dairy products has also facilitated cultural exchange. Cheese-making traditions from various countries have spread, leading to the production of diverse cheese varieties in regions where they were not traditionally made.

Economic Impact: The dairy trade has significant economic implications for both exporting and importing countries. It can drive economic growth in dairy-producing nations, create jobs, and provide a source of income for farmers. In importing countries, it ensures a stable supply of dairy products, even when local production is insufficient to meet demand.

Challenges and Controversies: The global dairy trade is not without challenges and controversies. Trade policies, tariffs, and subsidies can have a substantial impact on the dairy industry. Additionally, concerns about sustainability, animal welfare, and the impact of trade on local farmers and communities are subject to debate.

Dairy Security: The concept of dairy security has gained prominence as countries aim to ensure a consistent and adequate supply of dairy products to meet their population's nutritional needs. This has led to discussions about domestic dairy production and import policies.

Future Trends: The dairy trade continues to evolve with changing consumer preferences and dietary trends. The demand for dairy alternatives, like plant-based milks and cheeses, is influencing trade patterns and presenting new challenges and opportunities for the dairy industry.

The Family Farm Tradition

Even as dairy farming has evolved into an industrialized practice, the tradition of the family farm has remained a cornerstone of the industry. This chapter will celebrate the enduring spirit of family-owned dairies and the vital role they continue to play in local communities.

The family farm tradition is a cornerstone of dairy farming, and it holds a special place in the hearts of many individuals and communities. Despite the evolution of dairy farming into more industrialized practices, family-owned and operated dairies continue to thrive and play a vital role in local communities. Here are some reasons to celebrate the enduring spirit of family-owned dairies:

Heritage and Legacy: Many family-owned dairies have a rich heritage, passed down through generations. These farms often represent a deep connection to the land and a commitment to preserving agricultural traditions.

Local Community Support: Family farms are often deeply integrated into their local communities. They provide jobs, support local businesses, and participate in community events and initiatives. They are not just sources of milk but also centers of social and economic life.

Quality and Tradition: Family farms often prioritize the quality of their products. They may use traditional farming methods and take pride in producing high-quality milk, cheese, and other dairy products.

Environmental Stewardship: Many family-owned dairies prioritize sustainable and environmentally friendly practices. They have a vested interest in preserving the land for future generations and often implement practices that reduce their environmental footprint.

Animal Welfare: Smaller family farms often have a more hands-on approach to animal care. They can pay closer attention to the well-being of their livestock and may prioritize humane and ethical treatment of animals.

Local Food Movement: The resurgence of interest in locally sourced and farm-fresh food has benefited family-owned dairies. Consumers seek out local dairy products, supporting these small businesses.

Diversity of Dairy Products: Family farms are known for their artisanal and specialty dairy products. They often produce unique cheese varieties, yogurt, and other dairy items that cater to local tastes and preferences.

Educational Opportunities: Many family farms open their doors to the public, offering educational tours and events. This helps bridge the gap between consumers and the source of their food.

Resilience and Adaptability: Family farms are often nimble and adaptable. They can make changes to their operations or introduce new products based on consumer demand and market trends.

Sense of Belonging: Family-owned dairies often create a sense of belonging and community. Employees and customers may feel like part of an extended family, fostering loyalty and trust.

Cultural and Artistic Contributions: Some family farms integrate art and culture into their operations. For example, they might host art exhibitions or cultural events on the farm, enriching the local cultural landscape.

Preservation of Open Space: Family farms contribute to preserving open spaces and landscapes, making them important for biodiversity and scenic beauty.

Cultural Shifts and Dietary Trends

As we move through history, we'll also examine the impact of cultural shifts and dietary trends on the dairy industry. From wartime rations to the rise of vegetarianism and lactose intolerance awareness, we'll see how dairy has adapted to changing times.

Cultural shifts and dietary trends have had a significant impact on the dairy industry, shaping consumer preferences and influencing product development and marketing strategies. Here's how various shifts and trends have influenced the dairy industry throughout history:

Wartime Rations: During times of war and food shortages, rationing affected the availability of dairy products. Dairy farmers and manufacturers adapted by producing alternatives like dehydrated milk, which could be shipped to troops overseas. This experience highlighted the importance of dairy in the diet and encouraged dairy consumption when rationing ended.

Low-Fat and Diet Fads: In response to concerns about heart health, dietary fat, and weight management, there was a shift towards low-fat and fat-free dairy products. This led to the development of reduced-fat milk, yogurt, and cheese. However, concerns about the health benefits of whole dairy products have emerged in recent years, leading to a resurgence in their popularity.

Lactose Intolerance Awareness: Awareness of lactose intolerance has grown, leading to the development of lactose-free and lactose-reduced dairy products. These products provide options for individuals who have difficulty digesting lactose.

Vegetarianism and Veganism: The rise of vegetarianism and veganism has driven demand for dairy alternatives like almond milk, soy milk, and plant-based cheeses. Dairy companies have responded by expanding their product lines to include dairy-free options to cater to these dietary preferences.

Cultural Dietary Preferences: Dairy consumption varies significantly across cultures. Some cultures have a long tradition of dairy consumption, while others rely more on plant-based sources of nutrition. The dairy industry has adapted by producing products that align with cultural dietary preferences.

Functional Foods: There is a growing interest in functional foods, including dairy products fortified with probiotics, omega-3 fatty acids, and other health-enhancing ingredients. These products cater to consumers looking for specific health benefits from their food.

Organic and Sustainable Dairy: An increasing number of consumers are seeking organic and sustainably produced dairy products. This has led to the growth of organic dairy farming and products, as well as initiatives to reduce the environmental impact of dairy production.

Globalization and Fusion Cuisine: The globalization of food culture has resulted in the fusion of cuisines and flavors. This has encouraged innovation in dairy products, such as the incorporation of global flavors and ingredients in cheeses and yogurts.

Health and Wellness Trends: Consumers' awareness of health and wellness has influenced the dairy industry. There is a focus on incorporating probiotics and beneficial bacteria into products, as well as promoting the role of dairy in bone health and muscle recovery.

Clean Label and Transparency: Consumers are increasingly interested in the sources and ingredients of their food. The dairy industry has responded by emphasizing transparency, clean label products, and the use of fewer additives in dairy foods.

Convenience and Snacking: Busy lifestyles have driven the popularity of convenient dairy products like yogurt cups and single-serve cheeses. Dairy companies have adapted by creating on-the-go and snack-sized options.

Sustainable Packaging: There is a growing emphasis on environmentally friendly packaging for dairy products, with the industry exploring alternatives to single-use plastics and reducing waste.

Environmental and Sustainability Challenges

To provide a comprehensive view of the history of dairy farming, we must acknowledge the environmental challenges it has faced. This chapter will discuss the historical and contemporary concerns related to land use, water resources, and greenhouse gas emissions, shedding light on the ongoing efforts to make dairy farming more sustainable.

The history of dairy farming includes a range of environmental and sustainability challenges that have become increasingly important as the world grapples with climate change, resource conservation, and environmental preservation. Here, we'll explore some of the key issues and efforts related to sustainability in the dairy industry:

Land Use and Deforestation: Historically, the expansion of dairy farming has led to deforestation and land conversion, which can result in habitat loss, biodiversity decline, and increased greenhouse gas emissions. Sustainable dairy farming practices seek to limit deforestation and promote responsible land use.

Water Resources: Dairy farming requires significant water resources for both animal hydration and crop irrigation. Excessive water usage and improper waste management can lead to water pollution and depletion. Sustainable practices aim to reduce water use and protect water quality.

Greenhouse Gas Emissions: The dairy industry is a notable source of greenhouse gas emissions, primarily methane from enteric fermentation in cattle and manure management. Efforts to reduce emissions include improving feed efficiency, implementing methane capture systems, and exploring alternative feeds.

Animal Welfare: The ethical treatment of dairy cows is an important aspect of sustainability. Ethical concerns include issues related to confinement, access to pasture, and the use of growth hormones and antibiotics. Sustainable dairy farming prioritizes animal welfare and well-being.

Sustainable Feeding Practices: Dairy farmers are exploring more sustainable feeding practices, such as using byproducts from other industries, like citrus pulp, brewer's grains, and distillers grains, to reduce the environmental footprint of feed production.

Waste Management: Proper manure management is crucial for mitigating environmental impacts. Sustainable dairy farming includes responsible handling of manure, which can be converted into valuable resources like fertilizer and biogas.

Energy Efficiency: The energy demands of dairy farming, from milk cooling to milking machines, can be significant. Farms are adopting energy-efficient technologies and renewable energy sources to reduce their carbon footprint.

Sustainable Packaging: Dairy products are increasingly being packaged in environmentally friendly materials, such as recyclable and compostable packaging. Reducing plastic use and waste is a priority for sustainability.

Organic and Grass-Fed Dairy: Organic and grass-fed dairy farming practices promote sustainability by avoiding synthetic chemicals, promoting pasture-based systems, and supporting the welfare of dairy cows.

Certification Programs: Various certification programs, such as the USDA Organic label and the Certified Humane label, provide consumers with assurance that dairy products come from farms following specific sustainability and animal welfare standards.

Sustainable Supply Chains: Dairy companies are working to create sustainable supply chains, collaborating with farmers to adopt best practices and reduce the environmental footprint of dairy production.

Consumer Education: Many dairy producers are engaged in educating consumers about the importance of sustainable farming practices and how their choices can support a more sustainable dairy industry.

Milestones in Dairy Farming

Throughout this historical journey, we'll highlight key milestones that have defined the dairy industry. These may include the establishment of the first dairy cooperatives, the creation of quality standards and certifications, and the development of dairy farming schools and research institutions that have contributed to the industry's growth.

The history of dairy farming is marked by several key milestones that have shaped the industry and contributed to its growth and development. Here are some significant milestones in the history of dairy farming:

Domestication of Cattle: The domestication of cattle, which began around 10,000 years ago, marked the dawn of dairy farming. Early agricultural societies recognized the value of cattle for their milk and other products.

Introduction of Milking Techniques: Over time, techniques for milking cattle and processing milk evolved. Innovations like clay pots and later wooden buckets and milking stools made milking more efficient.

Development of Cheese: The art of cheesemaking has ancient origins, with evidence of cheese production dating back over 7,000 years. Cheese allowed for the preservation of milk and was an important source of nutrition in many cultures.

Medieval European Monasteries: In medieval Europe, monasteries played a crucial role in advancing dairy farming and cheese production. Monks often developed and improved cheesemaking techniques.

18th-Century Innovations: The 18th century saw significant advancements in dairy farming, including the development of the cream separator and the butter churn. These innovations improved milk processing and the production of butter.

Establishment of Dairy Cooperatives: The 19th century saw the rise of dairy cooperatives, like the cooperative creamery movement in Denmark. These cooperatives helped small-scale farmers pool their resources and improve the quality of dairy products.

Pasteurization: The 19th century also saw the discovery and development of pasteurization by

Louis Pasteur. This process significantly improved the safety and shelf life of dairy products.

Dairy Schools and Research: Dairy schools and research institutions, such as the Cornell University College of Agriculture and Life Sciences and the Babcock Dairy Center at the University of Wisconsin-Madison, were established in the late 19th and early 20th centuries. These institutions contributed to advancements in dairy science, technology, and education.

Dairy Quality Standards and Certification: The development of quality standards and certifications, like the USDA Grade A Pasteurized Milk Ordinance and organic dairy certifications, helped ensure the safety and quality of dairy products.

Growth of Industrial Dairy Processing: The 20th century witnessed the growth of industrial dairy processing, with the establishment of large-scale dairy processing plants and the production of various dairy products on a mass scale.

Genetic Advancements: Advances in animal genetics, such as selective breeding and artificial insemination, have led to the development of high-yield dairy cattle breeds like the Holstein and Jersey.

Sustainable Practices: The 21st century has seen a growing emphasis on sustainable dairy farming practices, including organic farming, improved waste management, and reduced environmental impact.

Global Dairy Trade Networks: The dairy industry has become a part of global trade networks, with countries exporting and importing dairy products to meet consumer demand.

Health and Nutrition Research: Ongoing research has expanded our understanding of the nutritional benefits of dairy products, leading to the promotion of dairy as a source of essential nutrients.

Consumer Trends: Changing consumer preferences, such as the rise of plant-based dairy alternatives, have spurred innovation in the dairy industry, leading to the development of new products and dairy alternatives.

Dairy Farming Traditions Around the World

Dairy farming traditions are not universal; they vary across countries and regions. This chapter will delve into the unique practices and customs associated with dairy farming in different parts of the world. From Alpine dairies in Switzerland to vast cattle ranches in the American Midwest, we'll explore the diversity of approaches to dairy farming.

Dairy farming traditions around the world reflect the unique landscapes, climates, cultures, and histories of different regions. Here's a glimpse into some of the diverse dairy farming practices and customs found in various parts of the world:

Alpine Dairies in Switzerland: Switzerland is known for its Alpine dairies, where cows are grazed in high-altitude meadows during the summer months. Cheesemakers in the Swiss Alps produce famous cheeses like Emmental and Gruyère. The tradition of transhumance, or moving cattle to high mountain pastures, is a vital part of Swiss dairy farming.

Gaucho Cattle Ranches in Argentina: In Argentina, vast cattle ranches, known as estancias, are home to traditional Gaucho cowboys who manage large herds of cattle. These cattle ranches produce milk for dairy products and are also known for their beef production.

French Cheese-Making: France is renowned for its cheese-making traditions, with each region producing its unique varieties. French dairy farms, particularly in Normandy, are famous for their dairy cows, like the Normande breed, which produces milk for Camembert and Brie cheeses.

Indian Dairying Practices: India has a long history of dairy farming, with the sacred cow being an integral part of Indian culture. The practice of dairy farming in India is diverse, with small-scale family farms as well as larger commercial operations. Milk is a crucial part of the Indian diet and is used to make products like ghee, paneer, and various sweets.

Mongolian Nomadic Dairying: In Mongolia, nomadic herders raise yaks and horses and produce dairy products like airag (fermented mare's milk) and aaruul (dried curd snacks). The harsh climate and nomadic lifestyle have shaped unique dairy farming practices.

New Zealand's Grass-Based Dairy: New Zealand is known for its extensive grass-based dairy farming. The country's dairy cows primarily graze on pasture, and New Zealand exports dairy products worldwide, including milk powder, cheese, and butter.

Amish and Mennonite Dairy Farming: In the United States, the Amish and Mennonite communities have maintained traditional dairy farming practices. They often use horse-drawn equipment and emphasize sustainable, low-tech farming methods.

Japanese Wagyu Cattle: Japan is famous for its Wagyu cattle, known for their marbled beef. While the primary focus is on beef production, there is a dairy component as well, and some Wagyu are raised for their milk to produce premium ice cream and cheeses.

Northern European Dairy Farming: Countries like the Netherlands and Denmark are known for their efficient and highly productive dairy farming systems. Holstein cows are commonly raised for their high milk production.

African Dairy Farming: Dairy farming in Africa varies widely depending on the region. In some parts, nomadic herders rely on cattle, while in other areas, there are smallholder dairy farmers. There is also a growing emphasis on improving dairy productivity and sustainability in African agriculture.

Israeli Kibbutz Dairy Farms: Israel's kibbutzim, or collective communities, have a strong tradition of dairy farming. The farms often prioritize technology and cooperative principles to maximize milk production and product quality.

Icelandic Skyr Production: Skyr is a traditional Icelandic dairy product similar to yogurt. Skyr is made from skimmed milk and has been a staple in Icelandic cuisine for centuries. Its production involves traditional bacterial cultures, resulting in a unique taste and texture.

The Dairy Farmer’s Way of Life

To provide a more personal perspective, we will share stories and anecdotes from dairy farmers and their families, offering a glimpse into the challenges they faced, their passion for their work, and the deep connections they maintain with their animals and the land.

The dairy farmer’s way of life is often deeply rooted in tradition, hard work, and a strong connection to the land and their animals. Here are some stories and anecdotes that offer a glimpse into the lives of dairy farmers and their families:

Morning Milking Ritual: For many dairy farmers, the day begins before dawn with the sound of cows lowing in the barn. They start the morning milking ritual, a daily routine that requires dedication and precision. Farmers often form strong bonds with their cows and know them by name. Each cow has its own personality, and over time, farmers develop a deep understanding of their needs and preferences.

Generational Farms: Many dairy farms have been passed down through generations. The love for the land and the commitment to continuing the family legacy run deep. These farms become not just places of work but also homes with a rich history and a sense of continuity.

Seasonal Rhythms: Dairy farming is often attuned to the seasonal rhythms of nature. Farmers eagerly await the arrival of spring when the pastures turn green and cows can graze outside. In the winter, they face the challenges of keeping the animals warm and well-fed. The changing seasons also influence the types of dairy products produced.

Adapting to Challenges: Dairy farmers are resilient in the face of challenges. Whether it's dealing with unpredictable weather, fluctuating milk prices, or disease outbreaks, they find ways to adapt and persevere. The sense of stewardship for their animals and the land drives them to overcome obstacles.

Family Involvement: The involvement of family members is often central to dairy farming. Children grow up learning the ropes and taking on responsibilities. The farm becomes a place of learning, hard work, and shared experiences. Families take pride in the tradition they uphold.

Community Support: Dairy farming is not just a job; it's a way of life that is often tightly knit with the local community. Neighbors lend a hand during busy times, and local businesses, like feed stores and equipment suppliers, play an essential role in sustaining the farm.

Innovation and Technology: While dairy farming traditions endure, modern farmers also embrace innovation and technology. Milking machines, automated feeding systems, and data-driven farm management tools have become essential to improve efficiency and productivity.

Quality over Quantity: Many small-scale dairy farmers prioritize the quality of their products over quantity. They take pride in producing artisanal cheeses, yogurts, and other dairy items that reflect their commitment to craftsmanship.

Challenges and Rewards: Dairy farming comes with its fair share of challenges, including long hours, physical labor, and financial uncertainties. Yet, the rewards are numerous, from the satisfaction of producing nutritious food to the deep sense of connection to the land and animals.

Sustainability and Conservation: Many dairy farmers are stewards of the land, implementing sustainable practices to protect the environment. They take measures to reduce their carbon footprint, improve waste management, and conserve natural resources.

Dairy Farming as an Economic Engine

Beyond its role in feeding people, dairy farming has been a significant economic force. We will discuss how it has contributed to rural economies, providing livelihoods for countless individuals and supporting local businesses.

Dairy farming has indeed been a significant economic engine, playing a vital role in supporting rural economies and providing livelihoods for countless individuals. Here are some of the key ways in which dairy farming contributes to local and regional economies:

Job Creation: Dairy farming provides employment opportunities in rural areas. These jobs extend beyond just the farm; they include positions in processing plants, distribution, transportation, and retail. In some communities, dairy farming is the primary source of employment.

Agricultural Infrastructure: Dairy farming contributes to the development of agricultural infrastructure. The need for facilities like barns, milking parlors, and silos supports local construction and manufacturing businesses.

Feed Production: Dairy farms create demand for feed crops such as alfalfa, corn, and soybeans. This stimulates local agriculture and generates income for crop farmers.

Equipment and Technology: Dairy farms invest in a range of equipment and technology, from tractors to milking machines and data management systems. This boosts the local economy by supporting equipment manufacturers and technology providers.

Supporting Small Businesses: Dairy farms require various goods and services, including veterinary care, feed suppliers, equipment repair, and transportation services. These businesses benefit from the steady clientele provided by dairy farming.

Tourism and Agritourism: Some dairy farms engage in agritourism activities, welcoming visitors for tours, farm stays, and events. These activities can boost the local tourism industry and create new sources of revenue.

Value-Added Products: Dairy farming is not just about milk; it includes the production of value-added products like cheese, yogurt, and ice cream. These products are often produced locally and sold directly to consumers or through local businesses.

Land Values and Property Taxes: Dairy farming can contribute to increasing land values in rural areas, which, in turn, impact property taxes and local government revenues. While this can be a double-edged sword for some, it does help support local services.

Community Contributions: Dairy farmers and their families are often active members of their communities. They participate in local organizations, contribute to charitable causes, and support community development initiatives.

Rural Development: Dairy farming can be a catalyst for rural development. As farms grow and expand, they can bring in new residents and businesses, potentially revitalizing rural areas.

Diversification: Dairy farming often leads to diversification of the local economy. For example, dairy communities may see the development of cheese shops, ice cream parlors, and other retail outlets specializing in dairy products.

Export Opportunities: In regions with surplus dairy production, dairy exports contribute to the national economy. Countries like New Zealand and the United States are major exporters of dairy products, earning foreign exchange and supporting the national balance of trade.

Looking Ahead: The Future of Dairy Farming

The chapter will also offer a glimpse into the future of dairy farming. How will emerging technologies, changing consumer preferences, and sustainability concerns shape the industry in the coming years? This will set the stage for later chapters that explore the current landscape and the path forward for dairy farming.

The future of dairy farming is marked by several emerging trends and challenges, as well as opportunities for growth and innovation. Here's a glimpse into what the future may hold for the dairy industry:

Sustainability and Environmental Stewardship: Sustainability will continue to be a focal point for the dairy industry. Farmers will explore more sustainable practices, from improving resource use to reducing greenhouse gas emissions. Sustainable packaging and waste reduction will also gain importance.

Technology and Automation: Dairy farms will increasingly adopt advanced technologies and automation. Robotics will play a significant role in milking, feeding, and monitoring animal health. Data-driven farm management will become more prevalent, enhancing efficiency and productivity.

Genomic Advancements: Genomic technologies will continue to influence dairy farming. This includes the use of genetic markers to select for desirable traits in dairy cattle, such as milk yield, disease resistance, and feed efficiency.

Plant-Based and Alternative Dairy Products: The rise of plant-based and alternative dairy products is expected to continue. Dairy companies will diversify their product lines to include dairy alternatives to cater to changing consumer preferences.

Consumer Focus on Health and Nutrition: As consumers become more health-conscious, dairy products will need to adapt. This may involve the development of functional dairy products enriched with probiotics, omega-3 fatty acids, and other health-enhancing ingredients.

Diversity of Dairy Products: The dairy industry will continue to innovate and expand its product range. This includes artisanal and specialty dairy products, as well as new flavor profiles and ingredient combinations to meet evolving consumer tastes.

Global Market Expansion: The global dairy trade will continue to grow as countries export and import dairy products to meet consumer demand. The industry will adapt to changing trade dynamics and market opportunities.

Climate-Resilient Farming: Climate change will bring new challenges to dairy farming, including extreme weather events and shifting weather patterns. Farmers will need to implement climate-resilient practices and technologies.

Education and Training: The future of dairy farming relies on the education and training of the next generation of farmers. Agricultural institutions and programs will play a crucial role in preparing individuals for modern dairy farming practices.

Ethical and Welfare Concerns: Consumer concerns about animal welfare will continue to shape dairy farming practices. Farmers will need to adhere to high standards of animal care and transparent practices.

Traceability and Transparency: Consumers will demand greater transparency in the dairy supply chain. Blockchain and other traceability technologies may be used to provide consumers with detailed information about the source and production of dairy products.

Diversification of Income Streams: To enhance financial stability, dairy farms may diversify their income streams. This could include agritourism, on-farm retail, and additional non-dairy agricultural activities.

Adaptation to Dietary Trends: Dairy farming will adapt to dietary trends, including the growth of lactose-free products and the increasing popularity of dairy products as ingredients in health-focused diets.

The Role of Dairy Farming in Feeding Populations

Throughout history, dairy farming has played a crucial role in providing sustenance to growing populations. This chapter will delve into the role of dairy as a source of essential nutrients, particularly protein and calcium, and its contribution to improved public health and nutrition.

Dairy farming has indeed played a crucial role in feeding populations and improving public health and nutrition in many parts of the world. Here's how dairy has been a source of essential nutrients and contributed to the well-being of communities:

Protein Source: Dairy products are a rich source of high-quality protein, containing all the essential amino acids needed for human health. Milk, cheese, and yogurt have been important protein sources, especially in areas where access to other protein-rich foods is limited.

Calcium and Bone Health: Dairy is one of the best dietary sources of calcium, a mineral vital for the development and maintenance of strong bones and teeth. Consuming dairy products, such as milk and yogurt, has been associated with reduced risk of osteoporosis and fractures.

Vitamins and Minerals: In addition to calcium, dairy products provide essential vitamins and minerals, including vitamin D, vitamin B12, riboflavin, and phosphorus. These nutrients are critical for various bodily functions and overall health.

Growth and Development: Dairy products are particularly important for the growth and development of children and adolescents. They provide the necessary nutrients for physical and cognitive development.

Improved Nutrition: The inclusion of dairy in diets has been associated with improved overall nutrition. Dairy products offer a balance of macronutrients (protein, fat, and carbohydrates) and micronutrients, contributing to a well-rounded diet.

Staple Food in Many Diets: In some regions, dairy products are a staple food, providing a significant portion of daily caloric intake. For example, cheese and yogurt are dietary staples in many Mediterranean and Middle Eastern countries.

Nutrient-Dense Options: Dairy products are nutrient-dense, meaning they provide a high concentration of essential nutrients relative to their calorie content. This makes them an efficient and valuable source of nutrition.

Affordability and Accessibility: Dairy products are often affordable and readily accessible to a wide range of populations, making them an essential part of the diet for many people.

Food Security: Dairy farming contributes to food security by providing a reliable source of nutrient-rich food. Dairy products are less susceptible to price fluctuations and spoilage compared to some other agricultural products.

Cultural and Culinary Significance: In many cultures, dairy products have cultural and culinary significance. They are essential ingredients in traditional dishes and cuisines, connecting people to their heritage and history.

Emergency Food Aid: In times of crisis, such as natural disasters and humanitarian emergencies, dairy products like milk powder are often included in food aid programs to address malnutrition and provide essential nutrition to vulnerable populations.

Dietary Diversity: Dairy products contribute to dietary diversity, helping to meet the nutritional needs of diverse populations with varying dietary preferences and restrictions.

Public Health Initiatives: Public health programs and campaigns have promoted the inclusion of dairy in diets, recognizing its role in supporting overall health and nutrition.

Dairy Farming and Land Use

The historical interaction between dairy farming and the land is a story of stewardship, sustainability, and the preservation of landscapes. We'll discuss how dairy farming has shaped landscapes, influenced land use policies, and even sparked conservation efforts in some regions.

The relationship between dairy farming and land use is a complex and evolving story of stewardship, sustainability, and the preservation of landscapes. Here's an exploration of how dairy farming has shaped landscapes, influenced land use policies, and even sparked conservation efforts in various regions:

Pasture-Based Farming: Traditionally, dairy farming has been closely tied to pasture-based systems, where cows graze on natural or cultivated grasslands. These pasture systems have a relatively low environmental footprint and promote biodiversity.

Land Management: Dairy farmers have been responsible for the stewardship of vast tracts of land. They manage pastures, invest in soil health, and adopt sustainable land management practices to maintain the productivity of the land over time.

Conservation Easements: In some regions, dairy farmers have partnered with conservation organizations to protect agricultural land from development. Conservation easements are legal agreements that restrict land use, preserving it for agriculture and open space.

Wetland Preservation: Dairy farms often have wetlands and water bodies on their properties. Preservation of these areas is important for wildlife habitat and water quality. Some farmers have implemented conservation practices to protect wetlands.

Manure Management: The responsible handling and management of manure are critical to avoid negative environmental impacts. Modern dairy farms employ strategies to recycle manure as a valuable resource for fertilizing crops.

Buffer Zones: To prevent nutrient runoff into water bodies, buffer zones of vegetation are often maintained around waterways and streams on dairy farms. These zones act as filters, protecting water quality.

Erosion Control: Dairy farming practices include erosion control measures, such as planting cover crops and maintaining grassed waterways, to reduce soil erosion and sedimentation.

Grassland Biodiversity: Pasture-based dairy farming systems can promote grassland biodiversity by providing diverse habitats for plants, insects, and wildlife.

Regulations and Zoning: Land use policies and regulations at the local, state, and national levels can influence where and how dairy farming can occur. Zoning regulations often designate areas for agricultural use, which can protect farmland from urban encroachment.

Agricultural Land Preservation: Some regions have implemented agricultural land preservation programs, protecting farmland from conversion to non-agricultural uses. These programs can support dairy farming by preserving available land.

Conservation Agriculture: Dairy farmers are increasingly adopting conservation agriculture practices, which emphasize minimal soil disturbance, crop rotation, and cover cropping to improve soil health and reduce environmental impacts.

Organic and Sustainable Farming: Organic and sustainable dairy farming practices place a strong emphasis on land stewardship. These systems prioritize soil health, reduce synthetic chemical use, and promote sustainable land use.

Community Efforts: Dairy farming communities often work together to protect the landscapes they rely on. They may engage in initiatives to conserve natural resources and promote sustainable land use.

Dairy in Mythology and Literature

To add an extra layer of depth, this chapter will also explore how dairy farming has been depicted in mythology and literature. From the Greek goddess Hera to the iconic literary references to milk and cheese, we'll uncover the rich symbolism and imagery surrounding dairy in human culture.

Dairy farming and dairy products have often been intertwined with symbolism, mythology, and literature in various cultures. Here's a glimpse into some of the ways dairy has been depicted in myth and literature:

1. Greek Mythology:

Hera, the Greek Goddess: In Greek mythology, Hera, the queen of the gods, was associated with cattle and the nurturing aspects of motherhood. She was often depicted with cows, emphasizing the connection between dairy and maternal care.

The Cattle of Helios: In the myth of the cattle of Helios, the sun god Helios had a herd of immortal cattle. These cattle were tended by his daughters and were associated with the life-giving and purifying qualities of the sun. The story underscores the symbolic importance of cattle and dairy in Greek mythology.

2. Hindu Mythology:

Kamadhenu: In Hindu mythology, Kamadhenu, the divine cow, is often depicted as a miraculous, wish-fulfilling cow. She is considered the mother of all cows and is a symbol of abundance, nourishment, and the importance of cattle in Indian culture.

3. Literature:

Milk and Honey in the Bible: The Bible frequently references "a land flowing with milk and honey" as a metaphor for a rich and prosperous land. This phrase underscores the significance of milk and dairy products as symbols of abundance and fertility.

Shakespearean References: In Shakespeare's works, there are numerous references to milk, butter, and cheese. For instance, in "Henry IV, Part 2," Falstaff humorously says, "Let the sky rain potatoes, let it thunder to the tune of 'Green Sleeves,' hail kissing-comfits and snow eringoes; let there come a tempest of provocation, I will shelter me here." This reflects the common presence of dairy products in daily life and literature during Shakespeare's time.

Cheese in "The Wind in the Willows": In Kenneth Grahame's "The Wind in the Willows," the character Ratty famously extols the virtues of cheese. His appreciation for cheese as the "only thing worth living for" is a playful reflection of the culinary and cultural significance of dairy products.

"The Cheese Stands Alone": The nursery rhyme "The Farmer in the Dell" features a line, "The cheese stands alone," emphasizing the importance of cheese in traditional farming communities.

4. Cultural Symbols:

Dairies in Norse Mythology: In Norse mythology, there are references to dairies as sources of nourishment. The concept of dairies as places of abundance and nurturing is depicted in these stories.

Milk as a Symbol of Purity: In various cultures, milk is often used as a symbol of purity, innocence, and motherhood. It is associated with nurturing and life-giving qualities.

The symbolism and imagery of dairy products in mythology and literature often reflect their cultural and historical significance. Whether as symbols of abundance, nourishment, or purity, these depictions underscore the role of dairy in human culture and its deep connection to everyday life and spirituality.

Dairy Farming and the Modern World

As we approach the contemporary era, we'll examine how dairy farming has evolved to meet the demands of the modern world. We'll consider the integration of technology, changes in consumer preferences, and the growing concerns for sustainability and animal welfare.

Dairy farming has evolved significantly to meet the demands of the modern world, with changes influenced by technology, shifting consumer preferences, and growing concerns for sustainability and animal welfare. Here's how dairy farming has adapted to the contemporary era:

Technological Integration:

Automation: Dairy farms have embraced automation, with robotic milking systems, automated feeders, and sensors that monitor cow health and productivity. These technologies enhance efficiency and data-driven decision-making.

Data Analytics: Modern dairy farms use data analytics to track cow performance, optimize feeding, and improve overall farm management. Data-driven insights help farmers make informed decisions.

Sustainability Initiatives:

Environmental Stewardship: Dairy farms are implementing sustainable practices to reduce their environmental footprint. These efforts include efficient manure management, reduced water usage, and measures to lower greenhouse gas emissions.

Renewable Energy: Some farms are investing in renewable energy sources, such as solar panels and methane digesters, to reduce their reliance on non-renewable resources and lower operating costs.

Animal Welfare Focus:

Comfortable Housing: Dairy farms are adopting more comfortable housing systems for cows, including spacious barns, clean bedding, and ventilation systems that ensure the well-being of the animals.

Nutrition and Health: Farmers are paying increased attention to cow nutrition and health. They work with veterinarians and nutritionists to develop balanced diets and provide timely healthcare.

Transparency: Transparency in animal welfare practices is becoming increasingly important. Consumers and advocacy groups are pushing for greater visibility into how dairy cows are cared for.

Diversified Dairy Products:

Plant-Based Alternatives: As plant-based diets gain popularity, dairy farms are diversifying their product offerings to include plant-based milk, yogurt, and cheese alternatives.

Functional Foods: There is a growing market for functional dairy products that offer health benefits beyond basic nutrition, such as probiotic yogurts and fortified milk.

Local and Artisanal Production:

Craft Dairy Products: Smaller, artisanal dairy producers are gaining attention for their high-quality, specialty products. They often emphasize traditional methods and unique flavors.

Farm-to-Table: The farm-to-table movement has encouraged the consumption of local, sustainably produced dairy products. Farmers markets and direct-to-consumer sales have become more popular.

International Trade and Export:

Globalization: Dairy farming is increasingly globalized, with countries exporting and importing dairy products to meet consumer demand. This has led to complex trade dynamics and economic impacts.

Consumer Health and Dietary Trends:

Lactose-Free and Dairy-Free Options: As awareness of lactose intolerance grows, the dairy industry has responded with lactose-free and dairy-free options, including lactose-free milk and dairy-free cheese and yogurt.

Protein and Health Benefits: Dairy is marketed as a source of high-quality protein and nutrients, aligning with consumer preferences for healthier food choices.

Regulatory Changes:

Quality Standards: Dairy products are subject to strict quality and safety standards, and these regulations have evolved to meet modern food safety and quality requirements.

Dairy farming in the modern world is characterized by a blend of tradition and innovation. It has adapted to meet the diverse needs and preferences of consumers while embracing technology and sustainability practices to ensure the industry's continued relevance and viability. The dairy sector remains a significant contributor to the food supply chain and the global economy.

CHAPTER THREE

Moo-ving Milk: Dairy Cow Breeds

The success of the dairy industry relies on the remarkable diversity of dairy cow breeds that have been selectively bred over centuries. Each breed possesses unique characteristics that influence milk production, flavor, and composition. In this chapter, we embark on an exploration of the world of dairy cow breeds, understanding the fascinating and distinctive attributes that make them central to the dairy landscape.

Bovine Evolution and Domestication

To truly appreciate the diversity of dairy cow breeds, we begin by tracing the evolutionary history of cattle. We explore how these majestic creatures were domesticated thousands of years ago and how various breeds have evolved to meet the changing needs of humanity.

The evolution and domestication of cattle are essential aspects of understanding the diversity of dairy cow breeds. Here's an overview of the evolutionary history and domestication of cattle:

Bovine Evolution:

Wild Ancestors: The domestic cattle we know today, primarily Bos taurus (taurine cattle) and Bos indicus (zebu cattle), have wild ancestors. Bos primigenius, also known as the aurochs, is the wild progenitor of these domesticated cattle. The aurochs were large, wild bovines that roamed Europe, Asia, and North Africa.

Domestication: The domestication of cattle is believed to have occurred around 10,000 years ago. Early human societies started to keep and breed cattle for various purposes, including as sources of meat, milk, and labor.

Diversity of Dairy Cow Breeds:

Taurine Cattle (Bos taurus):

Holstein: Holsteins are known for their high milk production. They have distinct black-and-white coloration and are common in dairy farming, particularly in North America and Europe.

Jersey: Jersey cattle are small but highly efficient milk producers. They are renowned for their rich and creamy milk, and they are often reddish-brown in color.

Zebu Cattle (Bos indicus):

Brahman: Brahman cattle are well-adapted to hot and humid climates. They are known for their humps and loose, saggy skin, which helps them regulate body temperature.

Guzerat: Guzerat cattle are another zebu breed that excels in milk production. They have distinctive humps and are often used in crossbreeding programs to improve milk production in tropical regions.

Dual-Purpose Breeds:

Brown Swiss: Brown Swiss cattle are known for their versatility, providing both milk and beef. They are well-regarded for their milk's butterfat content.

Simmental: Simmental cattle are dual-purpose breeds that produce both milk and meat. They are known for their large size and distinctive red-and-white or black-and-white coloration.

Minor Dairy Breeds:

Ayrshire: Ayrshire cattle are medium-sized and known for their adaptability and good milk production. They are often reddish-brown and white.

Guernsey: Guernsey cows are prized for their rich, golden milk. They are medium-sized and have a reddish-brown and white coat.

Emerging Dairy Breeds: Some emerging dairy breeds and crossbreeds are developed to combine the best traits of various breeds, such as high milk production, disease resistance, and adaptability to different climates.

Holstein: The Black-and-White Icon

The Holstein breed, easily recognizable by its striking black-and-white pattern, is the most renowned dairy cow worldwide. We delve into the history and characteristics of Holsteins, including their exceptional milk production capabilities and their importance in industrialized dairy farming.

Holstein cattle, with their distinctive black-and-white coloration, are indeed the most renowned and iconic dairy cow breed worldwide. Let's delve into the history, characteristics, and significance of Holsteins in the dairy industry:

History:

Origin: Holstein cattle, also known as Holstein-Friesians, have their origins in the northern regions of the Netherlands, particularly in the province of Friesland. They are named after the region.

Early Development: The breed's development can be traced back to the late 19th century when systematic breeding programs were established to improve the cattle's milk production. Selective breeding efforts focused on increasing milk yield and improving the breed's conformation.

Characteristics:

Distinctive Coloration: Holsteins are instantly recognizable by their black-and-white coat pattern. Their bodies are predominantly white with black spots or patches, giving them a striking appearance.

Size: Holsteins are typically large cows with a strong and robust build. They have a straight profile, and their legs are strong and well-muscled to support their weight.

Milk Production: Holsteins are renowned for their exceptional milk production capabilities. They are among the highest milk-producing dairy cows, with an average milk yield of 22,000 to 23,000 pounds of milk per year in the United States. Some individual Holsteins have set records with even higher milk production.

Butterfat and Protein Content: While Holsteins are known for their high milk production, their milk often has a lower butterfat and protein content compared to some other dairy breeds. However, this milk is still valuable for a wide range of dairy products.

Temperament: Holsteins are generally known for their calm and docile temperament, making them easier to manage on dairy farms.

Adaptability: Holsteins are adaptable to various climates and management systems. They are commonly found in dairy farms across the world, from North America and Europe to Asia and beyond.

Longevity: Holsteins typically have a longer productive life than some other dairy breeds. With proper care and management, they can provide several lactations over their lifespan.

Significance in Dairy Farming:

Holsteins are of immense importance in the industrialized dairy farming sector for several reasons:

High Milk Production: Their exceptional milk production capabilities make Holsteins a primary choice for dairy farmers focused on maximizing milk yield.

Economical Value: Holsteins are valued for their economic significance. They can efficiently convert feed into milk, making them cost-effective for large-scale dairy operations.

Global Presence: Holsteins are a global breed, with a presence in many countries. They contribute significantly to the dairy industry's global milk supply.

Selective Breeding: Selective breeding programs for Holsteins aim to improve traits related to milk production, longevity, and conformation, ensuring the continuous enhancement of the breed.

Crossbreeding: Holsteins are often used in crossbreeding programs to improve milk production in other dairy cow breeds or to develop cows with desirable traits for specific climates and environments.

Jersey: Small but Mighty

Jerseys, with their warm brown coats and gentle demeanor, are known for their rich and creamy milk. We’ll explore the history of the Jersey breed, its role in producing high-fat milk, and its place in small-scale, artisanal dairies.

Jersey cattle are known for their small but mighty presence in the dairy industry. Here’s a closer look at the history, characteristics, and significance of Jersey cows in the world of dairy farming:

History:

Origin: Jersey cattle originated on the island of Jersey, one of the Channel Islands located in the English Channel, near the coast of France. The breed’s history can be traced back to the late 18th century.

Breeding History: Jersey cattle were developed through selective breeding efforts aimed at improving their milk production and quality. The small island’s limited land area influenced the size of the cattle, resulting in the smaller stature of Jersey cows compared to some other dairy breeds.

Characteristics:

Coloration: Jerseys are known for their warm reddish-brown coat, often referred to as "fawn" or "fawn and white." Their faces are white, and they may have white markings on their legs and tail.

Size: Jersey cattle are smaller in size compared to some other dairy breeds, with a more compact and elegant build. They are well-proportioned, with a gentle and refined appearance.

Milk Production: While Jersey cows are not the highest milk producers in terms of volume, they are renowned for the quality of their milk. Jersey milk is rich and creamy, with higher butterfat and protein content compared to many other dairy breeds. This makes it ideal for producing cheese, butter, and other dairy products.

Butterfat and Protein Content: Jersey milk typically contains a higher percentage of butterfat and protein, making it valuable for the production of specialty dairy products and for its use in cheesemaking.

Adaptability: Jerseys are adaptable to various climates and management systems. Their smaller size and calm temperament make them well-suited for small-scale and artisanal dairies.

Longevity: Jersey cows often have a longer productive life compared to larger dairy breeds, making them an economical choice for dairy farmers.

Significance in Dairy Farming:

Jersey cattle have a special place in the world of dairy farming, particularly in small-scale and artisanal dairies, for several reasons:

High-Quality Milk: Jerseys are prized for their rich and high-quality milk. The milk's superior butterfat and protein content are ideal for making premium dairy products, such as cheese, ice cream, and yogurt.

Small Farms and Niche Markets: Jersey cows are well-suited for small dairy farms and niche markets where high-quality and specialty dairy products are produced. Their adaptability and gentle temperament make them a favorite among artisanal dairy producers.

Consumer Demand: The demand for locally produced, high-quality dairy products has grown, and Jersey milk meets these demands for quality and sustainability.

Crossbreeding: Jersey cattle are sometimes used in crossbreeding programs to improve the butterfat content of milk from other dairy breeds.

Jersey cows are celebrated for their ability to produce rich and creamy milk that's highly valued by dairy artisans and consumers who appreciate the exceptional flavor and quality of dairy products made from Jersey milk. Their importance in the dairy industry extends beyond just milk production, as they contribute to the diversity and uniqueness of dairy offerings in local and global markets.

Guernsey: Beauty and Utility

Guernsey cows, prized for their reddish-brown and white coloration, have a legacy that combines beauty with functionality. We'll uncover the history of Guernsey cattle, their adaptability, and their contributions to milk and cheese production.

Guernsey cows are celebrated for their unique combination of beauty and utility in the world of dairy farming. Let's explore the history, characteristics, and significance of Guernsey cattle:

History:

Origin: Guernsey cattle, as their name suggests, originated on the island of Guernsey, one of the Channel Islands in the English Channel, near the coast of France. The breed's history can be traced back to the early 19th century.

Breeding History: Guernsey cattle were developed through selective breeding efforts to improve their milk production, adaptability, and conformation. The breed's unique reddish-brown and white coloration distinguishes them from other dairy breeds.

Characteristics:

Coloration: Guernsey cattle are known for their striking reddish-brown and white coat. Their coloration is often described as "fawn and white." They have white markings on their faces, legs, and tail.

Size: Guernsey cows are of medium size, with well-proportioned bodies. They are robust and hardy, making them adaptable to various climates and management systems.

Milk Production: Guernsey cows are valued for their milk production, which combines both quality and quantity. While their milk production is not as high in volume as some other dairy breeds, it is renowned for its butterfat content, making it suitable for cheese, butter, and premium dairy products.

Butterfat and Protein Content: Guernsey milk contains a higher percentage of butterfat and protein compared to the milk of many other dairy breeds. This gives it a creamy texture and a rich, full flavor, making it ideal for making specialty dairy products.

Adaptability: Guernsey cattle are known for their adaptability to a wide range of climates and management systems. Their hardiness and ease of management make them suitable for small-scale and large-scale dairy operations.

Longevity: Guernsey cows often have a longer productive life than some other dairy breeds. They can provide multiple lactations over their lifespan with proper care and management.

Significance in Dairy Farming:

Guernsey cattle have a unique place in the world of dairy farming, contributing to the production of high-quality dairy products for several reasons:

Milk Quality: The high butterfat and protein content in Guernsey milk make it a valuable resource for producing premium dairy items. It is ideal for cheese, butter, and other specialty dairy products that rely on rich and flavorful milk.

Adaptability: Guernsey cows‘ adaptability to various climates and management systems means they can be found on diverse dairy farms across the world, contributing to local and regional dairy production.

Cheesemaking: Guernsey milk is particularly prized for cheesemaking, where the high butterfat content enhances the texture and flavor of the cheese.

Crossbreeding: Guernsey cattle are sometimes used in crossbreeding programs to improve the butterfat content of milk from other dairy breeds, or to introduce their unique coloration into other herds.

Ayrshire: A Breed with Heritage

The Ayrshire breed, often distinguished by its reddish-brown coat adorned with white markings, has deep historical roots. We'll explore the origins of Ayrshires and their unique balance of milk production and hardiness in various climates.

Ayrshire cattle, known for their reddish-brown coats adorned with white markings, are a breed with deep historical roots and unique characteristics. Let's delve into the history, characteristics, and significance of Ayrshire cattle in the world of dairy farming:

History:

Origin: Ayrshire cattle have their origins in the County of Ayr in southwestern Scotland, from which they derive their name. The breed's history can be traced back to the late 18th century.

Breeding History: Ayrshire cattle were developed through selective breeding efforts aimed at creating a well-rounded dairy cow. The breeding goals included improving milk production, hardiness, and adaptability to diverse climates.

Characteristics:

Coloration: Ayrshire cattle are recognized for their reddish-brown coat, often described as "cherry" or "mahogany" red, adorned with white markings. They typically have white faces and legs.

Size: Ayrshire cows are of medium size, with a balanced and sturdy build. They are well-proportioned, making them well-suited for various climates and management systems.

Milk Production: Ayrshire cows are valued for their milk production, which offers a combination of both quantity and quality. They are not the highest milk producers in terms of volume, but they are known for their ability to efficiently convert feed into milk.

Adaptability: Ayrshire cattle are highly adaptable to diverse climates and management systems. Their hardiness and versatility make them suitable for a wide range of dairy farming environments.

Longevity: Ayrshire cows often have a longer productive life compared to some other dairy breeds. With proper care and management, they can provide multiple lactations over their lifespan.

Significance in Dairy Farming:

Ayrshire cattle hold significance in the world of dairy farming for several reasons:

Milk Production: Ayrshire cows are known for their well-balanced milk production, with a good combination of volume and quality. Their milk is ideal for producing a wide range of dairy products, including cheese, butter, and fluid milk.

Hardiness: The adaptability and hardiness of Ayrshire cattle make them suitable for various climates and farming systems. They can thrive in both pasture-based and confinement-based systems.

Disease Resistance: Ayrshire cattle are often recognized for their disease resistance and general robustness, which contributes to their longevity and lower healthcare costs.

Environmental Adaptability: Ayrshires can adapt to diverse environmental conditions, including both hilly and lowland regions, further enhancing their versatility.

Sustainable Farming: Their ability to efficiently convert feed into milk makes Ayrshire cattle an attractive choice for sustainable and pasture-based farming systems.

Ayrshire cattle, with their unique combination of reddish-brown coloration and adaptable qualities, are celebrated for their role in milk production and their ability to thrive in various farming environments. They represent a breed with a rich heritage and a continuing legacy in dairy farming.

Brown Swiss: The Mountain Breed

The Brown Swiss breed, known for its grayish-brown coloration, excels in both milk production and adaptability. We'll uncover how this breed has thrived in alpine regions and contributed to both milk and cheese production.

Brown Swiss cattle, with their distinctive grayish-brown coloration, are a breed known for excelling in both milk production and adaptability, particularly in alpine regions. Let's explore the history, characteristics, and significance of Brown Swiss cattle in the world of dairy farming:

History:

Origin: Brown Swiss cattle, also known as Braunvieh, have their origins in the Alpine regions of Switzerland. The breed's history can be traced back to the late 15th century.

Breeding History: Brown Swiss cattle have a long history of selective breeding aimed at enhancing their milk production, hardiness, and adaptability to mountainous terrain and varied climates.

Characteristics:

Coloration: Brown Swiss cattle are known for their grayish-brown to dark brown coat, which can appear almost black. They have a unique coloration that distinguishes them from many other dairy breeds.

Size: Brown Swiss cows are medium to large in size, with a strong and robust build. Their bodies are well-muscled and well-proportioned.

Milk Production: Brown Swiss cows are valued for their milk production, which combines good milk volume and quality. Their milk is suitable for a wide range of dairy products, including cheese, butter, and fluid milk.

Butterfat and Protein Content: The milk of Brown Swiss cattle typically contains a moderate to high percentage of butterfat and protein, making it versatile for various dairy processing applications.

Adaptability: Brown Swiss cattle are known for their adaptability to alpine regions and mountainous terrain. They thrive in environments where the forage may be limited, and they are well-suited for extensive grazing systems.

Longevity: Brown Swiss cows are often recognized for their longevity and productive life, which can result in multiple lactations over their lifespan with proper care and management.

Significance in Dairy Farming:

Brown Swiss cattle hold significance in the world of dairy farming for several reasons:

Milk Production: Brown Swiss cows are known for their well-balanced milk production, offering a combination of volume and quality. Their milk is prized for its suitability in cheese production, especially in alpine cheese varieties.

Adaptability: The breed's adaptability to mountainous and challenging environments makes it a valuable choice for dairy farmers in hilly and alpine regions, where other breeds may struggle.

Cheese Production: The milk of Brown Swiss cattle is ideal for cheesemaking, particularly for alpine cheese types such as Emmental, Gruyère, and Appenzeller.

Environmental Resilience: Their ability to thrive in mountainous and sometimes harsh climates underscores their role in sustainable and environmentally friendly dairy farming.

Brown Swiss cattle, with their unique coloration and versatility in milk and cheese production, are celebrated for their adaptability to alpine regions. They represent a breed with a rich heritage and a continuing legacy in dairy farming, particularly in mountainous terrains and challenging climates.

Milking Shorthorn: Versatile and Sturdy

The Milking Shorthorn breed, characterized by a range of coat colors, has a rich history of versatility. We'll learn how these cows have been valued for their dual-purpose nature, providing both milk and meat.

Milking Shorthorn cattle, known for their diverse range of coat colors, have a rich history of versatility in the world of dairy farming. Let's explore the history, characteristics, and significance of Milking Shorthorn cattle:

History:

Origin: Milking Shorthorn cattle have their origins in the northeastern regions of England, particularly in the counties of Northumberland and Durham. The breed's history can be traced back to the late 18th century.

Breeding History: Milking Shorthorn cattle were developed through selective breeding efforts that aimed to create a dual-purpose breed suitable for both milk and meat production. They are known for their adaptability to various management systems and climates.

Characteristics:

Coat Colors: Milking Shorthorn cattle exhibit a wide range of coat colors and patterns, which can include red, white, or roan (a mix of red and white). The breed's coat color variations are one of its distinguishing features.

Size: Milking Shorthorn cows are of medium size, with a well-balanced and sturdy build. They are known for their adaptability and versatility in different farming environments.

Milk Production: Milking Shorthorn cows are valued for their milk production, which offers a balance of both quantity and quality. Their milk is suitable for producing cheese, butter, and other dairy products.

Meat Production: In addition to milk production, Milking Shorthorn cattle are highly regarded for their meat production qualities. They are known for their well-marbled, flavorful beef.

Adaptability: Milking Shorthorn cattle are adaptable to various climates and management systems. They are known for their hardiness and versatility, making them suitable for diverse farming environments.

Longevity: Milking Shorthorn cows often have a productive life that allows for multiple lactations with proper care and management.

Significance in Dairy Farming:

Milking Shorthorn cattle hold significance in the world of dairy farming for several reasons:

Dual-Purpose Nature: Milking Shorthorn cattle are one of the few dual-purpose breeds, excelling in both milk and meat production. This makes them a valuable choice for farmers looking for versatility in their livestock.

Adaptability: The breed's adaptability to various climates and management systems allows them to thrive in a wide range of farming environments.

Sustainable Farming: Milking Shorthorn cattle are well-suited for sustainable and pasture-based farming systems, where their versatility and adaptability can be a valuable asset.

Heritage Breed: The breed's rich history and heritage make it a symbol of traditional and diversified farming practices.

Milking Shorthorn cattle are celebrated for their unique combination of coat colors and their ability to provide both milk and meat. Their adaptability and versatility make them an important breed in the world of dairy farming, particularly in situations where farmers seek a well-rounded and dual-purpose breed.

Other Notable Dairy Breeds

This section will introduce readers to additional dairy cow breeds, such as the Dutch Belted, Normande, and Fleckvieh. Each of these breeds has unique characteristics and regional significance in dairy production.

Introducing readers to additional dairy cow breeds beyond the more well-known ones is a great way to showcase the diversity of cattle in the world of dairy farming. Here are brief introductions to the Dutch Belted, Normande, and Fleckvieh breeds, each of which has its unique characteristics and regional significance in dairy production:

Dutch Belted:

Origin: The Dutch Belted, also known as Lakenvelder, originated in the Netherlands. They are named for their distinctive white belt-like band that encircles their midsection.

Coloration: Dutch Belted cows have a black head and a white body with the characteristic black belt. This coloration sets them apart from other breeds.

Size: They are medium-sized cows with a balanced build.

Milk Production: Dutch Belted cows are valued for their milk production. They produce high-quality milk that is suitable for a range of dairy products.

Adaptability: They are adaptable to various climates and management systems. Their unique appearance and historical significance make them a rare and interesting breed.

Normande:

Origin: Normande cattle originate from the Normandy region of France. They have a history dating back several centuries.

Coloration: Normande cows have a distinctive reddish-brown coat with white markings. Some individuals may have a roan appearance.

Size: They are medium to large cows with a sturdy build.

Milk Production: Normande cows are valued for both their milk and meat production. Their milk has good butterfat content, and they are known for producing flavorful beef.

Adaptability: Normande cattle are well-adapted to the Normandy region's coastal climate and are prized for their hardiness and adaptability.

Cheese Production: The milk of Normande cows is ideal for cheese production, particularly for renowned French cheeses like Camembert and Pont-l'Évêque.

Fleckvieh:

Origin: Fleckvieh, which means "spotted cattle" in German, is a breed that originated in the Alpine regions of Europe, primarily Austria and Germany.

Coloration: Fleckvieh cows are typically light to dark brown with white markings. They often have a spotted or mottled appearance.

Size: Fleckvieh cattle are of medium to large size with a strong and robust build.

Milk Production: Fleckvieh is a dual-purpose breed, excelling in both milk and meat production. They produce milk with moderate to high butterfat content.

Adaptability: Fleckvieh cattle are highly adaptable to alpine regions and mountainous terrain. They are known for their hardiness and adaptability to challenging environments.

Meat Production: The breed is valued for its meat quality, providing well-marbled beef that is flavorful and sought after.

Introducing these lesser-known dairy cow breeds offers readers a broader perspective on the diversity of cattle in the dairy industry. Each of these breeds has its unique qualities, adaptability to specific regions, and regional significance in dairy and beef production.

Breed Selection and Crossbreeding

The chapter will conclude by examining the factors that influence breed selection in modern dairy farming. It will also discuss the practice of crossbreeding to harness the strengths of different breeds and create cows that are well-suited to specific farming conditions and goals.

The chapter on breed selection and crossbreeding in modern dairy farming is a crucial aspect of managing dairy herds effectively and efficiently. Here, we'll explore the factors that influence breed selection and the practice of crossbreeding to create cows that are well-suited to specific farming conditions and goals.

Breed Selection in Modern Dairy Farming:

Milk Production Goals: Dairy farmers often start with defining their milk production goals. They may choose breeds that are known for high milk yields if their primary focus is maximizing milk production.

Milk Quality: Some farmers prioritize milk quality over quantity. For producing high-quality dairy products like cheese and butter, they may opt for breeds with higher butterfat and protein content in their milk.

Climate and Environment: Environmental conditions play a significant role in breed selection. Certain breeds are better adapted to hot and humid climates, while others thrive in cold or mountainous regions.

Disease Resistance: Some breeds exhibit higher disease resistance and overall robustness. These traits can be especially important for minimizing healthcare costs and ensuring the health of the herd.

Farm Size and Management: The size of the dairy farm and the management system in place can influence breed selection. Smaller farms may prefer smaller breeds, while larger commercial operations might opt for high-yielding breeds.

Dual-Purpose vs. Specialized Breeds: Farmers must decide whether they want a dual-purpose breed (meat and milk) or a specialized breed for specific production goals.

Local Tradition and Preferences: In some regions, there may be a tradition of using specific breeds. Local preferences and market demands can also influence breed selection.

Crossbreeding in Modern Dairy Farming:

Crossbreeding is a practice where cows of different breeds are mated to harness the strengths of each breed and create a more balanced, resilient, and productive animal. Here are some considerations for crossbreeding:

Hybrid Vigor: Crossbred cattle often exhibit hybrid vigor, also known as heterosis. This can result in improved health, fertility, and overall performance compared to purebred animals.

Customization: Crossbreeding allows farmers to customize their herds to meet specific needs. For example, they can combine the high milk production of one breed with the disease resistance of another.

Environmental Adaptation: Crossbreeding can help create cows that are well-suited to specific environmental conditions. For example, crossing a heat-tolerant breed with a high-yield breed can result in cows adapted to hot climates.

Reducing Inbreeding: Crossbreeding helps reduce inbreeding, which can lead to healthier and more productive animals.

Market Demand: Some crossbred cattle may be in higher demand in certain markets, and farmers can take advantage of this demand.

Continuous Improvement: Through careful crossbreeding, farmers can continuously improve their herds, selecting for the traits that are most important for their specific goals.

It's important for dairy farmers to work with animal geneticists and experts to make informed breed selection and crossbreeding decisions. These decisions can significantly impact the overall success and sustainability of a dairy operation, ensuring that it meets its production goals and remains adaptable to changing conditions.

The Role of Dairy Cow Breeds in Agriculture

In this section, we'll explore how the various dairy cow breeds have played essential roles in the agricultural landscape. We'll discuss their contributions to the economy, local communities, and the global dairy market. This is where readers will gain insight into the practical applications of different breeds.

The role of dairy cow breeds in agriculture is multifaceted and essential to the functioning of the agricultural landscape. Each breed contributes to the economy, local communities, and the global dairy market in distinct ways. Here, we'll explore the practical applications of different breeds and their contributions to the agricultural sector:

Holstein:

Milk Production Powerhouse: Holsteins are synonymous with high milk production. Their large, high-yielding udders make them critical to dairy farms focused on maximizing milk production.

Economic Contribution: Holsteins are a driving force in the dairy industry's economic contributions. They provide a significant share of the milk supply, which, in turn, fuels the production of a wide range of dairy products, from fluid milk to cheese and butter.

Jersey:

Specialty Dairy Products: Jerseys are known for their rich and creamy milk. They play a vital role in producing specialty dairy products such as artisanal cheese, premium ice cream, and yogurt.

Small-Scale Farming: Jerseys are well-suited for small-scale, family-owned dairy farms. Their adaptability and docile temperament make them a practical choice for local communities.

Guernsey:

High Butterfat Milk: Guernsey cows are prized for their milk's high butterfat content, making it ideal for cheese and butter production. Their unique coloration adds to the visual appeal of dairy farms.

Adaptability: Guernsey cattle's adaptability to diverse climates and terrain contributes to their role in various agricultural settings.

Ayrshire:

Adaptable Dairy Breed: Ayrshires are versatile and well-suited to various farming conditions, thanks to their adaptability and hardiness.

Cheese Production: Their milk is well-regarded for cheese production, contributing to the production of a range of cheeses in different regions.

Brown Swiss:

Alpine Farming: Brown Swiss cattle excel in mountainous and alpine regions. Their adaptability to challenging environments makes them crucial for dairy farming in hilly terrains.

Meat Production: Their well-marbled meat is flavorful and sought after, contributing to both dairy and beef sectors.

Milking Shorthorn:

Dual-Purpose Breed: Milking Shorthorns are a valuable dual-purpose breed. They provide milk and meat, making them versatile for various agricultural operations.

Sustainable Farming: Their adaptability and versatility are significant for sustainable and diversified farming practices.

Crossbreeding:

Hybrid Vigor: Crossbreeding harnesses hybrid vigor, leading to healthier and more productive animals. It's an important strategy for optimizing performance and resilience in dairy farming.

Customization: Crossbreeding allows farmers to create herds that are well-suited to specific environmental conditions and production goals, enhancing the flexibility and adaptability of dairy operations.

In the agricultural landscape, dairy cow breeds are instrumental in providing essential resources such as milk, cheese, butter, and beef. They also play a significant role in local economies, supporting the livelihoods of farmers and contributing to the global dairy market. The choice of breed is influenced by various factors, including production goals, climate, market demand, and regional traditions, highlighting the diversity and adaptability of the dairy industry.

The Impact of Selective Breeding

Selective breeding has played a crucial role in shaping the characteristics of dairy cow breeds. We'll examine the science and art of selective breeding, highlighting the advancements in genetic selection that have led to improved milk production and quality.

Selective breeding has been a fundamental tool in shaping the characteristics of dairy cow breeds and improving their milk production and quality. In this section, we will explore the science and art of selective breeding, highlighting the advancements in genetic selection that have transformed the dairy industry. Here are some key points to consider:

Advancements in Selective Breeding:

Scientific Understanding: Selective breeding is rooted in a deep understanding of genetics. As our knowledge of genetics has advanced, so too has our ability to select for specific traits in dairy cows. Genetic markers, genomics, and DNA testing have become powerful tools in the hands of breeders.

Milk Yield: One of the primary objectives of selective breeding in dairy cows has been to increase milk production. Over the years, this has involved selecting cows with higher milk yields and breeding them to pass on these traits to their offspring.

Milk Quality: Beyond quantity, the quality of milk has also been a focus of selective breeding. Traits like butterfat content, protein content, and somatic cell count are considered when selecting breeding candidates.

Health and Disease Resistance: Selective breeding has been used to improve the overall health of dairy cows. Resistance to diseases, such as mastitis, and general robustness have been traits of interest.

Fertility and Reproduction: Fertility is a critical factor in dairy farming. Advances in selective breeding have helped improve the reproductive efficiency of dairy cows.

Environmental Adaptation: Selective breeding has been used to develop breeds or crossbreeds that are well-suited to specific environmental conditions, whether it's hot and humid climates or cold mountainous regions.

Genetic Selection:

Pedigree Analysis: Pedigree analysis involves studying the family history of dairy cows to identify individuals with desirable traits. Cows with a history of high milk production, good health, and other favorable characteristics are selected for breeding.

Genomic Selection: Genomic selection relies on DNA analysis to predict an individual cow's genetic potential. It allows breeders to identify desirable traits early in an animal's life, even before it starts producing milk.

Selective Matings: Careful consideration is given to selecting which bulls and cows should be bred to produce the next generation. This involves assessing the genetic compatibility of potential mates.

Selective Breeding Programs: Many dairy breed associations and organizations have established selective breeding programs with the goal of improving the genetics of the breed. These programs may include the use of artificial insemination and embryo transfer to propagate superior genetics.

The impact of selective breeding in dairy farming has been profound. It has led to significant increases in milk production, improved milk quality, and overall herd health. This not only benefits farmers but also ensures a consistent and high-quality supply of dairy products for consumers.

As science and technology continue to advance, selective breeding will remain a cornerstone of dairy farming, contributing to the sustainability and efficiency of the industry while addressing emerging challenges such as environmental sustainability and animal welfare.

Breed Conservation and Preservation

As the dairy industry evolves, some lesser-known breeds are at risk of extinction. This section will focus on the efforts to conserve and preserve these unique breeds, emphasizing the importance of biodiversity in agriculture.

Breed conservation and preservation are critical efforts in the dairy industry, particularly for lesser-known breeds that are at risk of extinction. This section will shed light on the importance of conserving these unique breeds and maintaining biodiversity in agriculture. Here are key points to consider:

The Importance of Breed Conservation:

Genetic Diversity: Biodiversity in dairy cow breeds is vital for preserving a wide range of genetic traits and adaptations. Different breeds may have specific qualities that can be crucial for future challenges in agriculture.

Local Adaptation: Some breeds have developed unique adaptations to specific environmental conditions. Conserving these breeds can help maintain the resilience of dairy herds in various regions.

Historical and Cultural Significance: Many traditional and heritage breeds have deep cultural and historical connections to local communities. They represent a part of agricultural heritage and cultural identity.

Niche Markets: Some unique dairy products are associated with specific breeds. The conservation of these breeds supports niche markets for artisanal cheeses and specialty dairy products.

Conservation Strategies:

Breeding Programs: Establishing breeding programs that focus on endangered or rare breeds is crucial. These programs can include artificial insemination and embryo transfer to propagate valuable genetics.

Diversity in Herds: Promoting diversity within dairy herds by incorporating rare breeds can help preserve their genetics. Crossbreeding strategies may be used to maintain the breed's unique traits.

Educational Initiatives: Raising awareness about the importance of breed conservation and the cultural significance of rare breeds can garner support from the public, governments, and agricultural organizations.

Genetic Banks: Maintaining genetic banks, such as semen and embryo repositories, ensures that genetic material from endangered breeds is safeguarded for future use.

Market Opportunities: Developing markets for products associated with unique breeds, such as specialty cheeses, can create economic incentives for breed conservation.

Examples of Endangered Breeds:

Canadienne: The Canadienne, a Canadian breed, was once widely used for dairy production but is now endangered. Efforts are being made to preserve its genetics.

Red Poll: The Red Poll breed, known for its dual-purpose nature, is also facing conservation challenges due to its declining population.

Vaynol: The Vaynol breed, a small dual-purpose breed from the United Kingdom, is critically endangered. Conservation initiatives aim to prevent its extinction.

Cikta: The Cikta, native to Hungary, is a rare breed known for its hardiness. Conservation efforts are essential to maintain this breed's unique traits.

Global Initiatives:

International organizations and conservation groups, such as the Rare Breeds Survival Trust (RBST) in the UK and the American Livestock Breeds Conservancy (ALBC), work to conserve and promote rare and endangered breeds.

Government Support: Many governments offer financial incentives, grants, or subsidies to support breed conservation and biodiversity efforts in agriculture.

Conserving and preserving unique dairy breeds is not only about safeguarding genetics but also about preserving cultural heritage and ensuring the resilience of the dairy industry in the face of changing agricultural needs and challenges. Biodiversity in dairy farming is a valuable asset for the future, and these efforts are crucial for maintaining it.

Crossbreeding and Hybrid Vigor

The chapter will also touch on the practice of crossbreeding, where two different dairy cow breeds are bred to combine their favorable traits. Readers will gain an understanding of the concept of hybrid vigor, which can result in healthier and more productive cows.

Crossbreeding is a common practice in dairy farming where two different dairy cow breeds are intentionally bred to combine their favorable traits. This chapter will provide readers with an understanding of the concept of hybrid vigor, which can result in healthier and more productive cows. Here are the key points to consider in this chapter:

Crossbreeding in Dairy Farming:

Genetic Diversity: Crossbreeding introduces genetic diversity into dairy herds. By combining the genetics of two different breeds, it is possible to create cows with a broader range of traits and characteristics.

Hybrid Vigor: Hybrid vigor, also known as heterosis, is the phenomenon where crossbred animals outperform their purebred counterparts in various aspects. This can include improved health, fertility, and overall performance.

Balancing Traits: Crossbreeding allows dairy farmers to balance different traits in their herds. For example, they can combine the high milk production of one breed with the disease resistance of another.

Customization: Farmers can customize their herds to meet specific production goals and adapt to their environmental conditions. This flexibility is a key advantage of crossbreeding.

Sustainability: Crossbreeding can contribute to the sustainability of dairy farming by creating more resilient and adaptable herds. Crossbred cows may be better suited to changing environmental conditions.

Understanding Hybrid Vigor:

Heterosis Effect: Hybrid vigor results from the combination of diverse genetic material. This effect can manifest in various ways, such as increased milk production, improved calf survival, and better disease resistance.

Reduced Inbreeding: Crossbreeding reduces the risk of inbreeding, which can lead to health problems and decreased fertility. Heterosis helps overcome some of these issues.

Improving Productivity: Crossbred cows often exhibit improved reproductive performance, leading to shorter calving intervals and more efficient use of resources.

Longevity: Hybrid vigor can contribute to the longevity of dairy cows. Crossbred cows may have longer and more productive lives compared to purebred animals.

Successful Crossbreeding Strategies:

Understanding Breed Characteristics: Farmers should have a thorough understanding of the characteristics and strengths of the breeds they are working with to create effective crossbreeding strategies.

Selective Mating: Careful consideration is given to selecting which bulls and cows should be bred to achieve the desired traits in the offspring.

Genetic Evaluation: Advances in genetics and genomics have made it easier to evaluate the genetic potential of animals and make informed crossbreeding decisions.

Monitoring and Record-Keeping: It's essential to monitor the performance of crossbred animals and maintain accurate records to assess the success of crossbreeding programs.

Crossbreeding and the concept of hybrid vigor have a significant impact on the productivity, health, and sustainability of dairy herds. This chapter will help readers understand the science and practical applications of crossbreeding in dairy farming, emphasizing the potential benefits of combining diverse genetic backgrounds to create more resilient and productive cows.

Modern Challenges and Trends

In the modern era, dairy farming faces new challenges, from changing climate patterns to the demand for more sustainable practices. We'll discuss how dairy cow breeds are adapting to these challenges and evolving to meet the needs of a changing world.

In the modern era, dairy farming faces a range of new challenges and trends, from changing climate patterns to the growing demand for more sustainable practices. This chapter will explore how dairy cow breeds are adapting to these challenges and evolving to meet the needs of a changing world. Here are the key aspects to consider in this chapter:

Climate Change and Environmental Challenges:

Changing Weather Patterns: Dairy farming is influenced by shifting weather patterns, including extreme weather events, droughts, and changing seasons. Breeds adaptable to these changes are crucial.

Sustainability: Modern dairy farming must address sustainability concerns, including reducing greenhouse gas emissions, conserving water resources, and minimizing the environmental impact. Certain breeds and crossbreeds may be more suited to sustainable practices.

Heat Stress: Rising temperatures and heat stress pose challenges for dairy cows. Breeds with heat-tolerant traits are increasingly important in many regions.

Consumer Preferences and Market Trends:

Plant-Based Alternatives: The growing popularity of plant-based dairy alternatives has led to evolving consumer preferences. Dairy cow breeds may need to adapt to maintain their market share.

Artisanal and Specialty Products: There is a growing market for artisanal and specialty dairy products. Some breeds, such as Jerseys, are well-suited for producing high-quality, distinctive dairy goods.

Health and Welfare Considerations:

Antibiotic Reduction: The dairy industry is under pressure to reduce the use of antibiotics. Breeds with inherent disease resistance and good overall health are valued.

Animal Welfare: There is an increased focus on animal welfare, including housing conditions and access to outdoor areas. Breeds that thrive in more extensive and welfare-friendly environments are advantageous.

Technological Advancements:

Genomic Selection: Advances in genomics and DNA analysis have revolutionized selective breeding. Breeders can now make more accurate and informed decisions about the genetic potential of dairy cows.

Precision Farming: Technology and data-driven practices have transformed dairy farming. Certain breeds may be more adaptable to precision farming methods and automation.

Local and Regional Variation:

Cultural Preferences: Dairy products and breeds can be closely tied to local and regional cultures. Understanding and adapting to cultural preferences are essential for dairy farming success.

Niche Markets: Some regions have unique niche markets for specialty dairy products. Certain breeds are particularly well-suited to these markets.

Genetic Preservation and Biodiversity:

Conservation Efforts: The conservation of rare and endangered dairy breeds is essential for maintaining genetic diversity. These breeds may hold valuable traits for future challenges.

Crossbreeding for Resilience: Crossbreeding strategies can create herds that are more resilient and adaptable to changing conditions.

Future Prospects

The chapter will conclude by looking at the future prospects of dairy cow breeds. How will the industry continue to evolve, and what role will genetics and breeding play in ensuring a sustainable and resilient dairy sector?

The Holstein Debate

This section will also address the Holstein debate, exploring the ongoing discussion about the dominance of Holsteins in industrial dairy farming and the potential advantages of diversifying dairy cow breeds for environmental, economic, and animal welfare reasons.

"The Holstein Debate" is a significant and thought-provoking topic in the world of dairy farming. It explores the ongoing discussion about the dominance of Holsteins in industrial dairy farming and the potential advantages of diversifying dairy cow breeds for environmental, economic, and animal welfare reasons. Here are key points to consider in this section:

The Dominance of Holsteins:

High Milk Production: Holsteins are renowned for their exceptional milk production capabilities. Their large size, efficient conversion of feed to milk, and high milk yield have made them the primary choice for many industrial dairy operations.

Economic Considerations: The economic advantages of Holsteins are evident. Their high milk production contributes significantly to dairy farm profitability, making them the preferred choice for commercial dairies.

Market Demand: Holstein milk is widely used in the production of various dairy products. The uniformity and consistent quality of Holstein milk meet the demands of the dairy processing industry.

The Advantages of Breed Diversification:

Environmental Sustainability: Diversifying dairy cow breeds can have environmental benefits. Some breeds are better adapted to specific environmental conditions, which can reduce the environmental impact of dairy farming.

Resilience: Breed diversity can enhance the overall resilience of dairy herds. Crossbreeding and incorporating other breeds can result in cows that are more adaptable to changing weather patterns and disease resistance.

Animal Welfare: Some argue that breed diversification can contribute to improved animal welfare. Some breeds are better suited to extensive or pasture-based systems, which align with animal welfare principles.

Niche Markets: Specialty dairy products, including artisanal cheeses and premium milk, are in demand. Diversified breeds, such as Jerseys, can cater to niche markets seeking unique and high-quality dairy products.

Balancing the Debate:

Selective Breeding: Breeders can selectively breed Holsteins for specific traits while promoting diversity within dairy herds. This approach can balance high milk production with other important characteristics.

Crossbreeding: Crossbreeding Holsteins with other breeds can harness the strengths of both and create more adaptable and resilient cows.

Local and Regional Considerations: The debate should consider the unique needs of different regions. What works best in one area may not be suitable for another, and local and regional considerations should be taken into account.

The Future of Dairy Farming:

The Holstein debate is an important part of discussions about the future of dairy farming. The dairy industry is evolving to address environmental concerns, animal welfare, and changing consumer preferences. Balancing the advantages of high milk production with other considerations will play a key role in shaping the future of dairy farming.

The Role of Dairy Cow Breed Associations

Dairy cow breed associations have played a significant role in preserving and promoting specific breeds. We'll examine their contributions, including breed registry programs, genetic improvement initiatives, and breed promotion efforts.

Dairy cow breed associations play a crucial role in preserving and promoting specific breeds within the dairy industry. This section will delve into their contributions, which include breed registry programs, genetic improvement initiatives, and breed promotion efforts. Here are key points to consider in this chapter:

Breed Registry Programs:

Maintaining Pedigree Records: Breed associations are responsible for maintaining accurate pedigree records of individual animals within the breed. This ensures the integrity of breed lines and genetic heritage.

Registration and Certification: Associations oversee the registration and certification of purebred animals, verifying that they meet the breed's standard in terms of physical characteristics and genetic lineage.

Genetic Evaluation: Breed associations often provide genetic evaluation services, helping farmers make informed breeding decisions based on an animal's genetic potential.

Genetic Improvement Initiatives:

Selective Breeding Programs: Many breed associations have established selective breeding programs to improve the genetic traits of their breed. These programs may include the use of elite sires, artificial insemination, and embryo transfer.

Genomic Selection: Advancements in genomics have enabled more precise genetic selection. Breed associations use DNA testing and genomic information to identify superior animals for breeding.

Evaluation of Breeding Bulls: Associations evaluate and select superior breeding bulls based on genetic merit, health, and conformation, ensuring that the best genetics are propagated within the breed.

Breed Promotion and Education:

Marketing and Promotion: Breed associations promote their breed to dairy farmers, emphasizing the breed's strengths and benefits. This marketing can help boost the breed's popularity and demand.

Education: Associations often provide educational resources and support to farmers regarding breed-specific management, husbandry practices, and breeding strategies.

Participation in Shows and Events: Many breed associations organize and participate in dairy shows and events, showcasing the breed's excellence and giving breeders the opportunity to exhibit their animals.

Networking and Community Building:

Community Building: Breed associations create a sense of community among breed enthusiasts and provide a platform for networking, knowledge sharing, and collaboration.

Advocacy: Associations may advocate for the interests of their breed within the broader dairy industry, ensuring that the breed's unique characteristics and contributions are recognized and valued.

Support for Rare Breeds:

Conservation Efforts: Some breed associations focus on preserving and conserving rare and endangered breeds. They work to maintain genetic diversity and prevent breed extinction.

Promoting Niche Markets: Associations for heritage or specialty breeds help farmers tap into niche markets for unique dairy products, contributing to economic sustainability.

Research and Development:

Breed-Specific Research: Breed associations may sponsor or conduct research specific to their breed, including studies on genetics, health, and performance traits.

Standard Development: They may participate in developing and refining breed standards, which define the physical and genetic characteristics that define the breed.

Breed associations are essential components of the dairy industry, ensuring the continuity and genetic quality of specific dairy cow breeds. They also provide valuable resources, support, and advocacy for breed enthusiasts and farmers, contributing to the preservation, promotion, and improvement of dairy breeds in diverse ways.

The Future of Dairy Cow Breeds

The chapter will conclude with a look into the future of dairy cow breeds. It will explore the challenges and opportunities that lie ahead, as well as the potential for breed-specific niche markets and sustainability practices to shape the industry in the coming decades.

"The Future of Dairy Cow Breeds" is a forward-looking chapter that explores the challenges and opportunities that lie ahead for dairy cow breeds in the evolving dairy industry. It will consider the potential for breed-specific niche markets and sustainability practices to shape the industry in the coming decades. Here are key points to consider in this concluding chapter:

Sustainability and Environmental Concerns:

Reducing Environmental Footprint: Dairy farming will continue to face pressure to reduce its environmental impact. Breeds and breeding strategies that align with sustainable farming practices will be highly valued.

Adaptation to Climate Change: As climate patterns shift, the adaptability of dairy cow breeds to changing environmental conditions will become increasingly important.

Consumer Preferences and Market Trends:

Plant-Based Alternatives: The rise of plant-based dairy alternatives will drive changes in the dairy industry. Breed associations and dairy farmers may explore new markets and value-added products.

Specialty and Artisanal Products: Niche markets for specialty and artisanal dairy products will continue to grow. Some breeds, such as Jerseys, may play a central role in catering to these markets.

Technological Advancements:

Genomic Selection: Advances in genomics will further refine selective breeding practices, allowing for more precise genetic improvement.

Automation and Precision Farming: Technology-driven automation and precision farming methods will become more prevalent. Some breeds may be better suited to these systems.

Niche Markets and Unique Dairy Products:

Heritage Breeds: The conservation and promotion of heritage and rare dairy cow breeds will help maintain genetic diversity and provide opportunities for unique, traditional dairy products.

Regionally Distinct Products: Some regions may focus on producing dairy products with distinctive regional characteristics, leveraging the strengths of specific breeds.

Research and Development:

Breed Improvement: Ongoing research and development efforts will continue to enhance the genetic potential and health of dairy cow breeds.

Environmental Stewardship: Research will further explore practices that promote environmental stewardship in dairy farming, with some breeds being more environmentally friendly.

Conservation and Biodiversity:

Preserving Rare Breeds: Conservation efforts for rare and endangered breeds will be essential for maintaining genetic diversity and resilience in the face of changing agricultural challenges.

Public Awareness and Advocacy:

Educating Consumers: Raising public awareness about the importance of breed diversity and sustainability in dairy farming will be important for the future of dairy cow breeds.

Adaptation to Regional Needs:

Local Solutions: Dairy cow breeds will continue to adapt to meet regional and local needs, whether it's for specific environmental conditions, market preferences, or cultural considerations.

As the dairy industry evolves, the future of dairy cow breeds will be shaped by the interplay of sustainability, consumer preferences, technology, and the need for genetic diversity. Breed associations, dairy farmers, and stakeholders in the industry will play a pivotal role in guiding the future of dairy cow breeds to meet the challenges and opportunities that lie ahead.

CHAPTER FOUR

Milk Processing: From Raw to Refined

In the world of dairy, milk is the canvas upon which a myriad of culinary delights are created. To fully appreciate the journey of milk from the cow's udder to our tables, we must understand the intricate process of milk processing. This chapter takes readers on a fascinating voyage through the transformation of raw milk into a wide array of refined dairy products.

The Dairy Processing Journey Begins

The chapter commences by examining the journey of raw milk from the farm to the processing plant. It explores the importance of quality control and safety measures at every stage to ensure that the milk remains pure and wholesome.

"The Dairy Processing Journey Begins" is the starting point of the dairy processing chapter, where we delve into the journey of raw milk from the farm to the processing plant. This section emphasizes the importance of quality control and safety measures at every stage to ensure that the milk remains pure and wholesome. Here are the key aspects to consider in this chapter:

Milk Collection and Transport:

Milking Process: The chapter can begin by describing the milking process on the dairy farm, whether it's done by hand or with modern milking machines.

Quality Control: Emphasize the importance of maintaining high standards of hygiene and cleanliness during milking to prevent contamination.

Milk Storage: Discuss the temporary storage of milk on the farm and the use of bulk tanks to keep the milk at a low temperature to maintain its quality.

Transportation: Explain how the milk is collected from farms, including the use of tanker trucks, and the need for regular cleaning and sanitation of these transport vehicles.

Quality Control and Safety Measures:

Milk Testing: Describe the routine testing of milk for quality parameters, including temperature, somatic cell count, and bacterial content.

Farm Inspections: Highlight the importance of regular inspections and audits on dairy farms to ensure compliance with quality and safety standards.

Cold Chain Management: Emphasize the need to maintain a continuous cold chain to prevent bacterial growth and spoilage during transportation.

Regulatory Compliance: Discuss the regulatory standards and guidelines that must be adhered to during the milk collection and transport process.

Farm-to-Plant Traceability:

Traceability Systems: Explain how modern technology enables traceability from farm to processing plant, allowing for quick identification and resolution of any quality or safety issues.

Data Collection: Describe how data on milk quality, source farms, and transportation routes is recorded and analyzed to ensure quality control.

Ensuring Wholesome Milk:

Quality Assurance: Discuss the importance of a robust quality assurance program, including regular training for farm workers and drivers.

Health and Hygiene: Emphasize the role of health and hygiene practices in ensuring that milk remains pure and safe for further processing.

Sustainability Considerations:

Energy Efficiency: Mention efforts to reduce energy consumption and greenhouse gas emissions during milk transportation.

Environmental Impact: Discuss sustainability practices related to milk collection, such as reducing water usage and minimizing waste.

By focusing on the journey of raw milk from the farm to the processing plant, this chapter sets the stage for understanding the critical steps in dairy processing and the measures in place to maintain the quality, safety, and wholesomeness of the milk. It provides readers with insight into the meticulous processes that go into ensuring that the milk is a high-quality raw material for dairy products.

Pasteurization: The Heat of the Matter

Pasteurization, a cornerstone of milk processing, is explored in depth. Readers will understand the significance of this process in killing harmful pathogens while preserving the nutritional value of milk.

"Pasteurization: The Heat of the Matter" is a pivotal chapter that explores pasteurization, a cornerstone of milk processing. In this section, readers will gain an in-depth understanding of the significance of pasteurization in killing harmful pathogens while preserving the nutritional value of milk. Here are key points to consider in this chapter:

The Significance of Pasteurization:

Historical Context: Provide a brief historical overview of the development of pasteurization by Louis Pasteur and its early applications in the dairy industry.

Pathogen Elimination: Explain that one of the primary objectives of pasteurization is to eliminate harmful microorganisms, such as bacteria and pathogens, that may be present in raw milk.

Safety Assurance: Emphasize the role of pasteurization in ensuring the safety of dairy products, which is crucial for public health and preventing foodborne illnesses.

The Pasteurization Process:

Heat Treatment: Describe the pasteurization process, which involves heating milk to specific temperatures and holding it at those temperatures for a predetermined period.

Temperature and Time Combinations: Explain that different pasteurization methods, such as high-temperature short-time (HTST) and low-temperature long-time (LTLT), use specific temperature and time combinations to achieve pasteurization.

Effect on Pathogens: Clarify how pasteurization works by denaturing the proteins and destroying the cellular structures of pathogens, rendering them harmless.

Preservation of Nutritional Value: Highlight that pasteurization is designed to minimize the loss of milk's nutritional value, such as vitamins, while achieving pathogen reduction.

Regulatory Standards:

Regulatory Oversight: Discuss the regulations and standards in place to ensure that pasteurization processes are carried out correctly and that dairy products meet safety requirements.

Heat-Resistant Pathogens: Explain that pasteurization doesn't eliminate all microorganisms, particularly heat-resistant spore-forming bacteria, and that these are addressed through additional measures in the dairy industry.

Variations in Pasteurization:

Ultra-Pasteurization: Mention variations of pasteurization, such as ultra-pasteurization, which involves higher temperatures and longer holding times, and their applications in dairy products.

Raw Milk Cheese: Address the specific requirements for pasteurization in the production of raw milk cheese and the reasons for using raw milk in certain cheese varieties.

Consumer Perception and Preferences:

Raw vs. Pasteurized Milk: Explore the ongoing debate and consumer preferences related to raw milk consumption and the potential risks associated with it.

Quality Control and Monitoring:

Quality Assurance: Explain the importance of quality control and monitoring in the pasteurization process, including the use of equipment to ensure precise temperature control.

Testing and Validation: Mention the routine testing and validation procedures that ensure the pasteurization process's effectiveness.

Continuous Innovation:

Emerging Technologies: Discuss the continuous innovation in pasteurization methods and technologies, including techniques such as ultra-high temperature processing (UHT) and microfiltration.

Non-Thermal Technologies: Explore non-thermal pasteurization methods, like high-pressure processing (HPP) and pulsed electric field (PEF) treatment, and their potential impact on the industry.

By delving into pasteurization, this chapter equips readers with a comprehensive understanding of a critical process in milk processing. It highlights the dual role of pasteurization in ensuring the safety of dairy products and preserving their nutritional value, while also addressing evolving technologies and consumer considerations.

Homogenization: Balancing the Blend

The chapter delves into the art of homogenization, a process that ensures a uniform mixture of milk's components. Readers will grasp how this technique keeps cream from separating, enhancing the consistency of dairy products.

"Homogenization: Balancing the Blend" is a chapter that explores the art of homogenization, a critical process in dairy processing that ensures a uniform mixture of milk's components. In this section, readers will grasp how homogenization works to keep cream from separating and enhances the consistency of dairy products. Here are key points to consider in this chapter:

The Importance of Homogenization:

Cream Separation: Explain that raw milk is an emulsion, with fat globules naturally separated from the other components, causing cream to rise to the top. Homogenization prevents this separation.

Enhanced Consistency: Emphasize that homogenization creates a consistent texture and flavor in dairy products, contributing to consumer satisfaction.

The Homogenization Process:

Principles of Homogenization: Describe the basic principles of homogenization, which involve breaking down fat globules into smaller sizes and distributing them evenly throughout the milk.

High Pressure: Explain that homogenization typically uses high-pressure pumps or homogenizers to achieve the desired particle size reduction.

Impact on Fat Globules: Clarify how the process affects fat globules, reducing their size and preventing them from reuniting.

Uniform Distribution: Highlight that the result of homogenization is a more uniform distribution of fat, which enhances the consistency and creaminess of dairy products.

Impact on Flavor and Texture:

Flavor Enhancement: Discuss how homogenization contributes to a smoother and more consistent flavor in dairy products, particularly in products like ice cream and milk.

Texture Improvement: Explain the impact of homogenization on the texture of dairy products, including the creaminess and mouthfeel.

Regulatory Considerations:

Regulations and Standards: Mention that regulatory bodies often establish standards and guidelines for homogenization processes to ensure product consistency and quality.

Variations and Innovations:

High-Pressure Homogenization: Explore variations and innovations in homogenization methods, such as high-pressure homogenization, which can offer advantages in certain applications.

Non-Dairy Applications: Discuss the application of homogenization in non-dairy products, such as fruit juices and cosmetics.

Consumer Preferences:

Natural vs. Homogenized: Address the debate regarding consumer preferences for homogenized vs. non-homogenized (cream-top) dairy products and the influence of health perceptions.

Quality Control and Monitoring:

Quality Assurance: Explain the importance of quality control and monitoring in the homogenization process to achieve the desired particle size distribution.

Testing and Validation: Mention the routine testing and validation procedures used to ensure that homogenization effectively prevents cream separation.

Sustainability Considerations:

Energy Efficiency: Discuss efforts to improve the energy efficiency of homogenization processes and their impact on sustainability in the dairy industry.

By exploring the science and art of homogenization, this chapter provides readers with a comprehensive understanding of how this process contributes to the consistency, flavor, and texture of dairy products. It also touches on consumer preferences, innovations, and sustainability efforts related to homogenization in the dairy industry.

Separation and Skim Milk Production

Readers will gain insight into how the separation process extracts cream from milk, leading to the creation of skim milk and a variety of cream products. This section explores the implications of separating milk components for different dairy products.

"Separation and Skim Milk Production" is a chapter that provides readers with insight into how the separation process extracts cream from milk, leading to the creation of skim milk and a variety of cream products. This section delves into the implications of separating milk components for different dairy products. Here are key points to consider in this chapter:

The Separation Process:

Principles of Separation: Describe the principles of separation, which typically involve the use of centrifugal separators that exploit the differences in density between cream and skim milk.

Cream Extraction: Explain how the separation process results in the extraction of cream, leaving behind skim milk.

Milk Composition: Discuss the composition of skim milk, which contains minimal fat but retains other milk components like proteins, lactose, and vitamins.

Skim Milk and Its Uses:

Nutritional Profile: Highlight the nutritional profile of skim milk, which is low in fat but rich in essential nutrients like protein, calcium, and vitamins.

Dairy Products: Explore the various dairy products that use skim milk as a key ingredient, such as yogurt, cheese, and low-fat dairy beverages.

Consumer Preferences: Discuss the reasons behind consumer preferences for skim milk, including health and dietary considerations.

Cream Products:

Types of Cream: Describe the different types of cream products that result from the separation process, including heavy cream, light cream, and half-and-half.

Applications: Explain the culinary and industrial applications of cream products in various dishes and food manufacturing processes.

Regulatory Standards:

Regulations and Standards: Mention that regulatory standards often specify the fat content and labeling requirements for different dairy products, including skim milk and cream.

Quality Control and Monitoring:

Quality Assurance: Explain the importance of quality control and monitoring in the separation process to ensure that cream and skim milk are produced within specified standards.

Testing and Validation: Mention the routine testing and validation procedures used to verify the fat content of cream and the fat-free nature of skim milk.

Sustainability Considerations:

Waste Reduction: Discuss sustainability efforts related to the reduction of waste and the repurposing of byproducts from the separation process.

Energy Efficiency: Explain how advances in separation technology have improved energy efficiency, reducing the environmental impact of the separation process.

By delving into the separation process and its implications for the creation of skim milk and cream products, this chapter provides readers with a comprehensive understanding of how this essential step in dairy processing influences the composition of various dairy products and meets consumer demands for both low-fat and cream-rich options.

The Craft of Cheese Making

This section of the chapter celebrates the art of cheese making. From curdling to curd formation and aging, readers will understand the intricacies of transforming milk into the countless varieties of cheese found around the world.

"The Craft of Cheese Making" is a section of the chapter that celebrates the art of cheese making. In this part, readers will gain insight into the intricacies of transforming milk into the countless varieties of cheese found around the world. Here are key points to consider in this section:

Introduction to Cheese Making:

Historical Perspective: Provide a brief historical overview of cheese making, including its ancient origins and development over time.

Variety of Cheeses: Emphasize the incredible diversity of cheese varieties found worldwide, shaped by different cultures, traditions, and local ingredients.

Key Stages of Cheese Making:

Curd Formation: Explain the process of curd formation, which involves coagulating milk and separating curds from whey. Different coagulation agents, such as rennet and acid, can be used.

Cutting and Draining: Describe the steps of cutting the curd and draining whey to achieve the desired texture and moisture content in the final cheese.

Salting: Explore the significance of salting cheese, which enhances flavor, texture, and preservation.

Molding and Pressing: Explain how curds are placed in molds and pressed to remove excess whey, shaping the cheese into its final form.

Aging and Ripening: Delve into the importance of aging and ripening cheese, which develops its flavor, aroma, and texture over time. Different aging conditions and methods result in a wide range of cheese varieties.

Cheese Categories:

Families of Cheese: Categorize cheeses into major families, such as soft cheese, semi-soft cheese, hard cheese, blue cheese, and fresh cheese. Provide examples and characteristics of each.

Artisanal and Industrial Cheese: Discuss the distinctions between artisanal and industrial cheese production, highlighting the craftsmanship and attention to detail in artisanal methods.

Regional and Cultural Influences:

Cheese Regions: Explore the influence of geographic regions on cheese styles, with examples of renowned cheese-producing areas like the French Alps, Italian countryside, and Swiss mountains.

Cultural Traditions: Describe how cultural traditions and practices have shaped unique cheese varieties and artisanal techniques.

Quality Control and Standards:

Quality Assurance: Explain the importance of quality control in cheese making, including milk quality, hygienic practices, and adherence to safety standards.

Appellations and AOCs: Discuss the concept of appellations and controlled designations of origin (AOCs), which protect and promote cheeses made in specific regions.

Sustainability Considerations:

Traditional and Sustainable Practices: Explore the sustainability of traditional cheese-making practices, such as using raw milk and natural fermentation.

Waste Reduction: Discuss efforts to minimize waste in cheese production and repurpose byproducts.

By celebrating the craft of cheese making, this section offers readers a deeper appreciation of the artistry, science, and culture that go into producing the world's diverse and delicious cheese varieties. It also highlights the influence of regional traditions and cultural heritage on cheese styles, as well as the significance of quality control and sustainability in the modern cheese-making industry.

Yogurt, Butter, and More

The chapter expands to encompass yogurt and butter production. Readers will learn about the fermentation process that yields yogurt's unique texture and flavor, and the churning and shaping of cream to create the beloved dairy delight—butter.

In the expanded chapter covering yogurt and butter production, readers will learn about the processes involved in creating yogurt and butter, two beloved dairy products with distinct characteristics. Here are key points to consider in this section:

Yogurt Production:

Fermentation Process: Describe the fermentation process in yogurt production, where beneficial bacteria (such as Lactobacillus bulgaricus and Streptococcus thermophilus) convert milk sugars into lactic acid, giving yogurt its tangy flavor and creamy texture.

Pasteurization and Homogenization: Explain the steps of pasteurizing and homogenizing milk to ensure safety and uniformity in yogurt production.

Starter Cultures: Discuss the importance of using specific starter cultures to initiate the fermentation process and achieve consistent yogurt quality.

Incubation and Fermentation: Detail the incubation period where milk is held at a specific temperature to allow bacterial activity, leading to yogurt formation.

Varieties and Additives: Highlight the various yogurt varieties, including Greek yogurt, flavored yogurts, and options with added fruit, honey, or other ingredients.

Health Benefits: Discuss the nutritional benefits of yogurt, including its probiotic content and contribution to gut health.

Butter Production:

Cream Separation: Explain that butter production begins with the separation of cream from milk, which can be achieved through natural separation or mechanical methods.

Churning: Describe the churning process, where cream is agitated to disrupt the fat globules, causing them to come together and form butter grains.

Whey Separation: Explain that the process also yields buttermilk as a byproduct, which can be used for other purposes.

Washing and Working: Discuss the washing and working of butter to remove excess buttermilk and achieve the desired texture.

Salt Addition: Mention the optional addition of salt to butter, which enhances flavor and acts as a preservative.

Types of Butter: Explore various types of butter, including sweet cream butter, cultured butter, clarified butter (ghee), and flavored butter.

Culinary and Baking Uses: Explain the culinary and baking applications of butter, from cooking and sautéing to pastry and cake making.

Quality Control and Standards:

Quality Assurance: Emphasize the importance of quality control in both yogurt and butter production, including milk quality, safety standards, and taste testing.

Regulatory Compliance: Mention that regulatory standards and labeling requirements apply to dairy products like yogurt and butter.

Sustainability Considerations:

Sustainable Practices: Discuss sustainable practices in dairy production, such as reducing waste and minimizing the environmental footprint of yogurt and butter manufacturing.

By covering yogurt and butter production, this section offers readers a comprehensive understanding of how these dairy products are made, their nutritional and culinary uses, and the importance of quality control and sustainability in the dairy industry. It also highlights the diversity of yogurt and butter varieties and their roles in various cuisines and cultures.

Condensed and Evaporated Milk

Readers are introduced to condensed and evaporated milk, products made by removing a significant portion of milk's moisture. This section explores the versatile uses of these dairy staples.

In the chapter covering condensed and evaporated milk, readers are introduced to these dairy products made by removing a significant portion of milk's moisture. This section explores the versatile uses of condensed and evaporated milk. Here are key points to consider in this section:

Introduction to Condensed and Evaporated Milk:

Production Process: Explain the common production process for both condensed and evaporated milk, which involves heating milk to reduce its moisture content and extend its shelf life.

Differences: Highlight the differences between condensed milk, which is sweetened, and evaporated milk, which is unsweetened.

Condensed Milk:

Sweetening: Describe the sweetening process involved in making condensed milk, typically with the addition of sugar or a sugar syrup during production.

Versatile Uses: Explore the wide range of culinary applications for condensed milk, including its use in desserts, baking, and beverage recipes.

Cultural and Global Significance: Discuss how condensed milk has played a significant role in various cultural and regional cuisines, particularly in desserts and sweet treats.

Evaporated Milk:

Unsweetened Nature: Explain that evaporated milk is unsweetened, making it a versatile ingredient for both savory and sweet dishes.

Cooking and Baking: Discuss the use of evaporated milk in cooking and baking, such as in sauces, soups, and creamy desserts.

Dilution and Reconstitution: Mention the practice of diluting evaporated milk with water to reconstitute it to a liquid state, similar to regular milk.

Health Considerations:

Nutritional Profile: Compare the nutritional profiles of condensed and evaporated milk with regular milk, highlighting their higher calorie content due to reduced moisture.

Lactose Content: Address the potential advantages of using evaporated milk for individuals with lactose intolerance, as it contains lower levels of lactose.

Quality Control and Standards:

Quality Assurance: Emphasize the importance of quality control in the production of condensed and evaporated milk, including safety standards and taste testing.

Regulatory Compliance: Mention that regulatory standards and labeling requirements apply to these dairy products.

Sustainability Considerations:

Sustainability Practices: Discuss sustainable practices in condensed and evaporated milk production, such as energy-efficient manufacturing and waste reduction.

By covering condensed and evaporated milk, this section offers readers a comprehensive understanding of these dairy staples, their versatile uses in cooking and baking, and their significance in various cuisines. It also addresses nutritional aspects and sustainability considerations related to the production of these dairy products.

Sweet Temptations: Ice Cream and Desserts

The chapter concludes with the sweet side of dairy processing, focusing on the production of ice cream and various desserts. Readers will be immersed in the world of freezing, flavoring, and creating the delectable treats that make dairy a source of indulgence.

In the concluding section of the chapter, which focuses on the sweet side of dairy processing, readers will be immersed in the world of freezing, flavoring, and creating delectable treats, including ice cream and various desserts. Here are key points to consider in this section:

Introduction to Ice Cream and Desserts:

Historical Perspective: Provide a brief historical overview of ice cream and dessert production, tracing their origins and evolution.

Diversity of Desserts: Highlight the incredible diversity of dairy-based desserts, including custards, puddings, gelatos, and more.

Ice Cream Production:

Ingredients: Explain the primary ingredients in ice cream production, including milk, cream, sugar, and flavorings.

Mix Preparation: Describe the preparation of the ice cream mix, which involves heating and blending the ingredients to create a uniform base.

Freezing Process: Detail the freezing process in ice cream makers, which incorporates air and results in the creamy texture of ice cream.

Flavoring and Inclusions: Explore the wide variety of flavors, mix-ins, and inclusions used in ice cream, ranging from classic vanilla to inventive combinations.

Packaging and Storage: Explain the packaging and storage of ice cream to maintain its quality and prevent ice crystals.

Dairy-Based Desserts:

Custards and Puddings: Describe the production of custards and puddings, which involve thickening milk or cream with eggs or starch.

Gelato: Discuss the making of gelato, an Italian-style ice cream that has a lower fat content and is served at a slightly higher temperature.

Toppings and Sauces: Explore the various toppings and sauces used to enhance the flavor and presentation of dairy-based desserts.

Cultural and Regional Desserts:

Global Influences: Highlight the influence of different cultures and regions on dairy-based dessert recipes, such as Italian tiramisu, French crème brûlée, and Indian kulfi.

Traditional Celebrations: Discuss how dairy desserts play a role in traditional celebrations and holidays worldwide.

Quality Control and Standards:

Quality Assurance: Emphasize the importance of quality control in ice cream and dessert production, including taste testing and ingredient sourcing.

Regulatory Compliance: Mention that regulatory standards and labeling requirements apply to dairy-based desserts.

Sustainability Considerations:

Sustainability Practices: Discuss sustainable practices in dairy dessert production, such as reducing waste and responsible sourcing of ingredients.

By concluding with a focus on ice cream and dairy-based desserts, this section provides readers with a delicious and indulgent perspective on dairy processing. It highlights the creativity in flavoring and presenting dairy desserts, the cultural and regional influences, and the importance of quality control and sustainability in producing these sweet delights.

Customization and Innovation in Milk Processing

Throughout the chapter, readers will gain an understanding of the customization and innovation taking place in the dairy processing industry. Modern techniques, from adding fortifications to meet specific nutritional demands to catering to diverse dietary preferences, are showcased.

The chapter on customization and innovation in milk processing showcases the modern techniques and advancements in the dairy processing industry, catering to diverse dietary preferences and specific nutritional demands. Here are key points to consider throughout this chapter:

Customization and Innovation in Milk Processing:

Consumer Preferences: Highlight the importance of understanding consumer preferences and dietary choices in shaping the dairy processing industry.

Fortification: Explain the practice of fortifying milk and dairy products with additional nutrients, such as vitamins, minerals, and probiotics, to meet specific nutritional demands.

Lactose-Free and Dairy Alternatives: Discuss the rise of lactose-free dairy products and the development of dairy alternatives like almond milk, soy milk, and oat milk to accommodate lactose intolerance and diverse dietary choices.

Plant-Based Innovations: Explore the innovations in plant-based dairy alternatives, including advancements in taste, texture, and nutrition.

Low-Fat and Low-Sugar Products: Discuss the creation of low-fat and low-sugar dairy products to align with health-conscious consumer preferences.

Reduced Environmental Impact: Address sustainability efforts in dairy processing, including reducing water usage, greenhouse gas emissions, and waste generation.

Customized Packaging: Explain how dairy products are now offered in various packaging options, such as single-serve containers, eco-friendly materials, and innovative designs.

Quality Assurance: Emphasize the importance of maintaining high-quality standards while customizing and innovating dairy products.

Regulatory Compliance:

Regulations and Labeling: Discuss the need to comply with regulations and labeling requirements while introducing new dairy products and innovations.

Collaborative Research and Development:

Industry Collaboration: Highlight the collaborative efforts between the dairy industry and research institutions to advance dairy processing techniques and develop innovative products.

Sustainability Considerations:

Environmental Responsibility: Discuss the commitment of the dairy industry to reduce its environmental footprint, from sustainable sourcing to energy-efficient processing.

By exploring customization and innovation in milk processing, this chapter provides readers with a comprehensive understanding of how the dairy industry adapts to changing consumer preferences and dietary needs. It also showcases the efforts to reduce environmental impact and the collaborative research and development initiatives that drive dairy processing innovation.

Sustainability and Environmental Considerations

The chapter will emphasize the increasing importance of sustainable practices in milk processing. Readers will explore how dairy processors are adopting environmentally friendly technologies and practices to reduce waste, save energy, and minimize their carbon footprint.

The chapter on sustainability and environmental considerations in milk processing emphasizes the increasing importance of sustainable practices in the dairy industry. Readers will explore how dairy processors are adopting environmentally friendly technologies and practices to reduce waste, save energy, and minimize their carbon footprint. Here are key points to consider in this chapter:

Importance of Sustainability:

Environmental Awareness: Highlight the growing awareness of environmental issues and the need for sustainable practices in dairy processing.

Consumer Expectations: Discuss how consumers are increasingly looking for sustainable and eco-friendly dairy products.

Sustainable Practices in Milk Processing:

Reducing Waste: Explain how dairy processors are implementing waste reduction strategies, such as minimizing byproducts and finding alternative uses for them.

Energy Efficiency: Describe the adoption of energy-efficient technologies and practices in dairy processing to reduce energy consumption and greenhouse gas emissions.

Water Conservation: Discuss water-saving initiatives in dairy processing, such as recycling and reusing water and reducing water usage.

Eco-Friendly Packaging: Highlight the use of sustainable and recyclable packaging materials in the dairy industry.

Sustainable Sourcing:

Responsibly Sourced Ingredients: Explain how dairy companies are increasingly sourcing ingredients and raw materials from sustainable and ethical suppliers.

Local Sourcing: Discuss the benefits of local sourcing, which reduces transportation-related emissions and supports local economies.

Renewable Energy: Explore the use of renewable energy sources, such as solar and wind power, in dairy processing facilities.

Carbon Footprint Reduction:

Carbon Neutral Initiatives: Describe efforts by dairy processors to achieve carbon neutrality by reducing emissions and offsetting the remaining carbon footprint.

Carbon Labeling: Discuss the adoption of carbon labeling on dairy products to inform consumers about their environmental impact.

Sustainability Certifications: Explain the importance of sustainability certifications, such as organic and Fair Trade, in dairy products.

Collaboration and Research:

Collaborative Efforts: Highlight collaborations between dairy industry stakeholders, research institutions, and environmental organizations to promote sustainability.

Regulatory Compliance:

Compliance with Environmental Regulations: Discuss the need for dairy processors to adhere to environmental regulations and standards.

By focusing on sustainability and environmental considerations in milk processing, this chapter provides readers with a comprehensive understanding of the efforts made by the dairy industry to reduce its environmental impact and promote eco-friendly practices. It also addresses the growing consumer demand for sustainable dairy products and the collaborative initiatives that drive sustainability in the dairy sector.

The Magic of Fermentation

Fermentation plays a pivotal role in the transformation of milk into a variety of dairy products. Readers will delve into the science and art of fermentation, understanding how beneficial bacteria and cultures are harnessed to craft products like sour cream, kefir, and probiotic yogurts.

In the chapter titled "The Magic of Fermentation," readers will delve into the science and art of fermentation, understanding how beneficial bacteria and cultures are harnessed to craft a variety of dairy products like sour cream, kefir, and probiotic yogurts. Here are key points to consider in this chapter:

Introduction to Fermentation:

Fermentation Defined: Define fermentation as a biological process in which microorganisms, such as bacteria and yeast, convert sugars into other compounds, often leading to changes in taste, texture, and preservation.

Historical Significance: Highlight the historical importance of fermentation in food preservation and flavor enhancement, including dairy products.

Microorganisms in Fermentation:

Beneficial Bacteria: Introduce the concept of beneficial bacteria, such as lactic acid bacteria (LAB), which are commonly used in dairy fermentation.

Yeast and Other Microbes: Mention the role of yeast and other microorganisms in specific dairy fermentation processes.

Fermentation in Dairy Products:

Yogurt Production: Explain the process of yogurt fermentation, where specific bacterial strains, including Lactobacillus bulgaricus and Streptococcus thermophilus, convert milk sugars into lactic acid, giving yogurt its distinctive tangy flavor and texture.

Sour Cream and Crème Fraîche: Explore the fermentation of sour cream and crème fraîche, which involves the use of LAB to thicken and acidify cream.

Kefir Fermentation: Discuss kefir production, which includes the use of kefir grains, a combination of LAB and yeast, to ferment milk, resulting in a probiotic-rich, effervescent beverage.

Probiotic Yogurts: Explain the emergence of probiotic yogurts, which contain specific live bacterial cultures known for their potential health benefits.

Cultural Significance:

Cultural and Regional Variations: Discuss how different cultures and regions have their own unique fermented dairy products, such as Indian dahi, Middle Eastern labneh, and Eastern European smetana.

Health Benefits and Probiotics:

Probiotics Explained: Define probiotics as live microorganisms that may provide health benefits when consumed in adequate amounts.

Gut Health: Discuss the potential positive effects of probiotics on gut health, digestion, and the immune system.

Quality Control and Standards:

Quality Assurance: Emphasize the importance of quality control in the fermentation of dairy products, ensuring the presence of the desired microbial strains and product consistency.

Regulatory Compliance: Mention that regulatory standards and labeling requirements apply to dairy products, especially those containing live cultures.

Sustainability Considerations:

Sustainable Fermentation Practices: Explore the use of sustainable practices, such as reducing waste and conserving energy, in dairy fermentation.

By delving into the magic of fermentation, this chapter offers readers a deeper understanding of the vital role microorganisms play in crafting a diverse array of dairy products. It also highlights the cultural and regional variations in fermented dairy products, the potential health benefits of probiotics, and the importance of quality control and sustainability in dairy fermentation processes.

From Milk to Cream

This section explores the creation of various cream-based products, including heavy cream, light cream, and half-and-half. It delves into the fat separation process that leads to different cream varieties and their culinary applications.

In the section titled "From Milk to Cream," readers will explore the creation of various cream-based products, including heavy cream, light cream, and half-and-half. This section delves into the fat separation process that leads to different cream varieties and their culinary applications. Here are key points to consider in this section:

Introduction to Cream Products:

Cream Defined: Define cream as the fat-rich component of milk, with variations in fat content, thickness, and culinary uses.

Importance of Fat Content: Explain the significance of fat content in cream products for achieving different textures and flavors in recipes.

Cream Separation Process:

Centrifugation: Describe the separation process of cream from milk, often achieved through centrifugation, which utilizes the difference in density between cream and milk.

Fat Content Adjustment: Explain how the fat content of cream can be adjusted by controlling the separation process and combining it with milk.

Varieties of Cream:

Heavy Cream: Define heavy cream as the cream with the highest fat content, typically around 36% or higher, and explain its thick and rich consistency. Explore its use in whipping, sauces, and desserts.

Light Cream: Describe light cream, which has a lower fat content than heavy cream but is still richer than milk. Discuss its culinary uses, including in coffee, soups, and baking.

Half-and-Half: Explain half-and-half, a mixture of equal parts milk and light cream, which offers a balance of creaminess and lower fat content. Discuss its common use in coffee and as a topping.

Culinary Applications:

Cooking and Baking: Discuss the application of cream products in various recipes, such as soups, sauces, custards, and pastries.

Whipping and Desserts: Explore how heavy cream is whipped to create whipped cream and used in a wide range of desserts like ice cream, mousse, and panna cotta.

Quality Control and Standards:

Quality Assurance: Emphasize the importance of quality control in cream production to maintain consistency in fat content and flavor.

Regulatory Compliance: Mention that regulatory standards and labeling requirements apply to cream products.

Sustainability Considerations:

Sustainable Practices: Discuss sustainable practices in cream production, such as reducing waste and minimizing the environmental impact.

By exploring the transformation of milk into cream products, this section provides readers with a comprehensive understanding of the variations in cream, their culinary applications, and the importance of quality control and sustainability in cream production. It also highlights the role of cream in enhancing the flavor and texture of a wide range of dishes and desserts.

Concentration and Dehydration

Readers will gain an appreciation for concentration and dehydration techniques, which are instrumental in producing dairy ingredients like milk powder and whey protein. These versatile ingredients find their way into numerous food products, from infant formula to sports nutrition.

In the section titled "Concentration and Dehydration," readers will gain an appreciation for concentration and dehydration techniques, which are instrumental in producing dairy ingredients like milk powder and whey protein. These versatile ingredients find their way into numerous food products, from infant formula to sports nutrition. Here are key points to consider in this section:

Introduction to Concentration and Dehydration:

Purpose and Significance: Explain the purpose and importance of concentration and dehydration techniques in dairy processing.

Diverse Applications: Highlight how the resulting dairy ingredients are used in a wide range of food products, both within and outside the dairy industry.

Concentration Techniques:

Evaporation: Describe the process of evaporation, where heat is applied to remove water from milk, resulting in a concentrated liquid.

Ultrafiltration: Explain ultrafiltration, a membrane-based technique that separates water and smaller molecules from larger molecules, concentrating the desired components.

Dehydration Techniques:

Spray Drying: Discuss the spray drying process, where liquid dairy products are atomized into fine droplets and exposed to hot air to remove moisture, resulting in powdered products.

Freeze Drying: Explain freeze drying, which involves freezing liquid dairy products and then subjecting them to a vacuum, causing the frozen water to sublimate, leaving behind freeze-dried powder.

Dairy Ingredients Produced:

Milk Powder: Detail the production of milk powder, which includes both skim milk powder and whole milk powder. Explain how they are used in reconstituted milk, bakery products, confectionery, and more.

Whey Protein Concentrate (WPC) and Isolate (WPI): Describe the production of whey protein concentrate and isolate, highlighting their applications in sports nutrition, infant formula, and functional foods.

Lactose: Mention the production of lactose from whey and its use in dairy products, infant formula, and pharmaceuticals.

Nutritional and Functional Benefits:

Long Shelf Life: Explain how concentration and dehydration contribute to extended shelf life for dairy ingredients.

Ease of Storage and Transport: Highlight the benefits of dairy ingredients in powdered form for ease of storage and transportation.

Quality Control and Standards:

Quality Assurance: Emphasize the importance of quality control in the production of dairy ingredients, including flavor, texture, and nutritional content.

Regulatory Compliance: Mention that regulatory standards and labeling requirements apply to dairy ingredients.

Sustainability Considerations:

Sustainable Practices: Discuss sustainable practices in dairy ingredient production, such as energy-efficient methods and waste reduction.

By exploring concentration and dehydration techniques in dairy processing, this section provides readers with a comprehensive understanding of how these processes are used to produce essential dairy ingredients. It also highlights the versatility of these ingredients in various food products, their nutritional and functional benefits, and the importance of quality control and sustainability in their production.

Flavoring and Aromatization

The art of flavoring and aromatization in milk processing is highlighted. Readers will explore how flavors are introduced to milk to create a wide range of flavored milk products, from chocolate milk to fruit-infused dairy beverages.

In the section on "Flavoring and Aromatization" in milk processing, readers will explore the art of introducing flavors to milk to create a wide range of flavored milk products, from chocolate milk to fruit-infused dairy beverages. Here are key points to consider in this section:

Introduction to Flavoring and Aromatization:

The Art of Flavor: Explain the significance of flavor in dairy products and how it influences consumer preferences.

Versatility of Milk: Highlight the versatility of milk as a base for creating a wide variety of flavored dairy products.

Flavoring Techniques:

Natural Flavor Sources: Discuss the use of natural sources for flavoring, such as fruit extracts, vanilla beans, and cocoa.

Artificial Flavorings: Explain the use of artificial flavorings, which can mimic the taste of various fruits, spices, and other natural sources.

Emulsions and Suspensions: Describe the need for emulsifiers and stabilizers to ensure that flavorings are evenly distributed in milk.

Common Flavored Milk Products:

Chocolate Milk: Explore the production of chocolate milk, which involves the addition of cocoa or chocolate syrup to milk.

Strawberry Milk: Discuss the flavoring process for strawberry milk, typically achieved using strawberry puree or flavoring agents.

Fruit-Infused Dairy Beverages: Explain how fruit flavorings are used to create fruit-flavored yogurts, smoothies, and dairy-based drinks.

Vanilla and Other Flavors: Mention the use of vanilla, spices, and other flavorings in dairy products like ice cream and custards.

Sensory Aspects:

Texture and Mouthfeel: Discuss how flavorings can affect the texture and mouthfeel of dairy products.

Aroma: Highlight the importance of aroma in flavor perception and how it can be influenced by flavorings.

Cultural and Regional Variations:

International Flavored Dairy Products: Explore how different cultures and regions have their own unique flavored dairy products and traditional recipes.

Health Considerations:

Sugar Content: Address the potential impact of added sugars in flavored milk products and the trend toward reduced sugar options.

Natural Flavor Trends: Discuss the growing demand for natural and clean-label flavorings in dairy products.

Quality Control and Standards:

Flavor Consistency: Emphasize the importance of maintaining consistent flavor profiles in flavored dairy products.

Regulatory Compliance: Mention that regulatory standards and labeling requirements apply to flavored dairy products.

Quality Control and Assurance

This section emphasizes the critical importance of quality control and assurance in milk processing. Readers will understand the stringent standards and testing procedures that ensure that dairy products meet safety and quality requirements.

In the section on "Quality Control and Assurance" in milk processing, readers will understand the critical importance of quality control and assurance in the dairy industry. This section emphasizes the stringent standards and testing procedures that ensure that dairy products meet safety and quality requirements. Here are key points to consider in this section:

Introduction to Quality Control and Assurance:

The Significance of Quality: Explain the essential role of quality control and assurance in dairy processing to ensure that dairy products are safe, consistent, and meet consumer expectations.

Safety and Quality Standards:

Regulatory Standards: Discuss the regulatory standards and guidelines set by government agencies to ensure the safety and quality of dairy products, such as the Food and Drug Administration (FDA) in the United States.

International Standards: Mention international organizations like the Codex Alimentarius, which establish global food standards, and their impact on dairy product quality.

Testing and Analysis:

Microbiological Testing: Explain the importance of microbiological testing to detect and control harmful pathogens and ensure product safety.

Chemical Analysis: Discuss chemical analysis methods to monitor factors like fat content, protein content, and lactose content in dairy products.

Sensory Evaluation: Highlight sensory evaluation techniques that assess the flavor, texture, appearance, and aroma of dairy products.

Nutritional Testing: Mention nutritional testing to determine the nutritional content of dairy products, including vitamins and minerals.

Allergen Testing: Explain allergen testing to detect the presence of common allergens like milk proteins in dairy products.

Quality Assurance in Dairy Processing:

Process Control: Describe process control measures to maintain consistent product quality, including temperature control, pasteurization, and packaging.

Good Manufacturing Practices (GMP): Discuss the importance of GMP in dairy processing facilities to maintain sanitary conditions and product integrity.

Hazard Analysis and Critical Control Points (HACCP): Explain the HACCP system, which identifies and addresses potential hazards at critical points in the production process.

Quality Standards for Specific Dairy Products:

Cheese: Discuss quality standards for cheese, including factors like flavor profiles, texture, and ripening.

Yogurt: Explore quality standards for yogurt, addressing aspects like acidity, viscosity, and flavor.

The Role of Dairy Ingredients in Food Manufacturing

Readers will gain insight into the integral role that dairy ingredients play in the broader food industry. The chapter will delve into how dairy components like casein, whey, and lactose are used in food manufacturing, from enhancing texture to providing nutritional value.

In the chapter on "The Role of Dairy Ingredients in Food Manufacturing," readers will gain insight into the integral role that dairy ingredients play in the broader food industry. The chapter will delve into how dairy components like casein, whey, and lactose are used in food manufacturing, from enhancing texture to providing nutritional value. Here are key points to consider in this chapter:

Introduction to Dairy Ingredients in Food Manufacturing:

The Versatility of Dairy Ingredients: Explain how dairy ingredients are used in various food products to enhance texture, flavor, and nutritional content.

Common Dairy Ingredients:

Casein: Discuss the use of casein, a protein derived from milk, in a wide range of food products, including cheese, processed meats, and bakery items, as a source of protein and as a texturizing agent.

Whey: Explore the applications of whey, a byproduct of cheese and yogurt production, in food manufacturing, such as in protein supplements, sports nutrition products, and baked goods.

Lactose: Explain how lactose, the natural sugar in milk, is used in food products as a sweetener and bulking agent, as well as in confectionery and pharmaceuticals.

Dairy Ingredient Functionality:

Texture Enhancement: Describe how dairy ingredients like casein and whey proteins are used to improve the texture, mouthfeel, and creaminess of food products.

Nutritional Enrichment: Highlight the nutritional value of dairy ingredients, such as their protein content and essential amino acids.

Emulsification: Discuss the emulsifying properties of dairy ingredients in creating stable and consistent food products, including dressings and sauces.

Flavor Enhancement: Explain how dairy ingredients can enhance the flavor profile of certain foods, such as dairy-based desserts and snack foods.

Food Categories Utilizing Dairy Ingredients:

Bakery and Confectionery: Explore how dairy ingredients are used in baking, including in bread, cakes, and cookies, and their role in confectionery products like chocolates and candies.

Dairy Alternatives: Discuss the use of dairy ingredients in dairy alternative products like plant-based milk and non-dairy desserts.

Protein Supplements: Explain the role of dairy ingredients, particularly whey protein, in protein supplements and sports nutrition products.

Processed Meats: Explore the applications of dairy ingredients, such as casein, in processed meat products like sausages and meat analogs.

Dairy-Based Beverages: Discuss how dairy ingredients are used in dairy-based beverages, including smoothies, flavored milk, and yogurt drinks.

Health and Nutritional Considerations:

Nutritional Benefits: Highlight the nutritional benefits of dairy ingredients, such as protein content, essential nutrients, and amino acids.

Lactose-Free Options: Discuss lactose-free alternatives and dairy ingredients suitable for lactose-intolerant individuals.

Packaging, Preservation, and Shelf Life

The chapter will also explore the significance of packaging, preservation, and extending shelf life in the dairy industry. Readers will learn about the various methods and technologies used to protect dairy products and ensure their longevity.

In the chapter on "Packaging, Preservation, and Shelf Life" in the dairy industry, readers will explore the significance of packaging, preservation, and extending shelf life in the dairy sector. The chapter will delve into the various methods and technologies used to protect dairy products and ensure their longevity. Here are key points to consider in this chapter:

Introduction to Packaging and Preservation:

Importance of Packaging: Explain the critical role of packaging in protecting dairy products from external factors, such as light, air, moisture, and contaminants.

Extending Shelf Life: Emphasize the importance of preserving dairy products to ensure their freshness and safety for an extended period.

Packaging Materials and Technologies:

Packaging Materials: Discuss the various packaging materials used in the dairy industry, including glass, plastic, cartons, and pouches.

Aseptic Packaging: Explain aseptic packaging, a method that involves sterilizing both the product and the packaging to extend shelf life without refrigeration.

Modified Atmosphere Packaging (MAP): Explore MAP, a technique that modifies the atmosphere inside the package to slow down product deterioration.

Vacuum Packaging: Discuss vacuum packaging, which removes air from the package to prevent oxidation and microbial growth.

Packaging for Different Dairy Products:

Fluid Milk: Describe the packaging methods for fluid milk, including bottles, cartons, and bags.

Yogurt and Dairy Desserts: Explain the packaging options for yogurt and dairy desserts, such as plastic cups and multi-packs.

Cheese: Discuss the packaging of cheese, which can vary from vacuum-sealed bags to wax coatings.

Butter and Spreads: Explore the packaging of butter and spreads, which may include tubs and foil-wrapped blocks.

Preservation Techniques:

Refrigeration: Explain the role of refrigeration in preserving dairy products, especially for perishable items.

Freezing: Discuss the freezing of dairy products, such as ice cream and frozen desserts, to maintain their texture and quality.

UHT (Ultra-High Temperature) Processing: Describe UHT processing, which involves heating dairy products to a very high temperature to achieve extended shelf life.

Challenges in Packaging and Preservation:

Environmental Impact: Address the environmental impact of packaging materials and the industry's efforts to reduce waste and improve sustainability.

Food Safety: Discuss the importance of maintaining food safety throughout the packaging and preservation process.

Quality Control and Assurance:

Quality of Packaging: Emphasize the need for quality control and assurance to ensure that packaging materials meet the required standards and regulations.

Expiration Dates: Explain how expiration dates are determined for dairy products to guarantee their safety and quality.

Sustainability Considerations:

Sustainable Packaging: Explore sustainable packaging practices, such as using recyclable materials and reducing single-use plastics.

Reducing Food Waste: Discuss how extended shelf life can contribute to reducing food waste.

By exploring the role of packaging, preservation, and shelf life in the dairy industry, this chapter provides readers with a comprehensive understanding of the methods and technologies used to protect dairy products and ensure their longevity. It also addresses the challenges in packaging and preservation, quality control and assurance, and the industry's commitment to sustainability in packaging practices.

The Journey Continues: From Processing Plant to Your Table

Readers will appreciate that the journey of milk processing doesn't end at the processing plant. The chapter will conclude by tracing the path of dairy products from the production facility to the consumer's table, highlighting the steps that ensure the products remain safe and enjoyable to the last spoonful.

In the chapter titled "The Journey Continues: From Processing Plant to Your Table," readers will appreciate that the journey of milk processing doesn't end at the processing plant. The chapter will conclude by tracing the path of dairy products from the production facility to the consumer's table, highlighting the steps that ensure the products remain safe and enjoyable to the last spoonful. Here are key points to consider in this chapter:

Introduction to the Journey from Processing Plant to Table:

Overview: Introduce the concept of the journey of dairy products from the processing plant to the consumer's table, emphasizing the importance of maintaining quality and safety throughout the distribution and consumption process.

Packaging and Distribution:

Packaging Preparation: Explain how dairy products are packaged at the processing plant to maintain freshness and quality.

Distribution Channels: Describe the various distribution channels, including refrigerated trucks, wholesalers, and retailers, that transport dairy products to consumers.

Retail Display and Storage:

Retail Handling: Discuss how dairy products are displayed and stored in grocery stores and supermarkets to maintain the cold chain and product integrity.

Consumer Selection: Explain how consumers select dairy products based on factors like expiration dates and visual inspection.

Transportation and Home Storage:

Consumer Transportation: Address the importance of consumers maintaining the cold chain during transportation, such as keeping dairy products in a cooler when shopping.

Home Storage: Offer guidelines for consumers on proper home storage of dairy products, including refrigeration and safe handling practices.

Safe Handling and Consumption:

Food Safety Awareness: Highlight the significance of food safety awareness among consumers and the importance of checking expiration dates.

Proper Handling: Emphasize proper handling practices at home, including avoiding cross-contamination and maintaining cold storage.

Sustainability Considerations:

Sustainable Practices: Discuss how sustainable packaging and transportation practices are incorporated into the journey of dairy products from plant to table.

Quality Control and Assurance Throughout:

Quality Control: Explain how quality control and assurance continue to be a priority throughout the journey of dairy products.

Consumer Experience:

Enjoyment and Satisfaction: Address the importance of consumers' enjoyment and satisfaction with dairy products, including taste and quality.

By tracing the path of dairy products from the processing plant to the consumer's table, this chapter provides readers with a comprehensive understanding of the steps and considerations involved in ensuring that dairy products remain safe, fresh, and enjoyable until they are consumed. It also emphasizes the role of sustainability, quality control, and proper handling practices in this journey.

CHAPTER FIVE

Milk: The Nutrient Powerhouse

Milk, often referred to as "nature's most perfect food," is a nutrient powerhouse that has been a dietary staple for centuries. In this chapter, we will delve deep into the nutritional value and health benefits of milk, understanding why it is hailed as a valuable source of essential nutrients.

Milk as a Complete Food

The chapter will commence by highlighting milk's role as a complete food source, providing a wide array of nutrients in a single package. Readers will explore how milk contains carbohydrates, proteins, fats, vitamins, and minerals, making it a valuable source of energy and nutrition.

Milk is often regarded as a complete food due to its rich and balanced nutritional composition. It provides a wide array of essential nutrients, making it a valuable source of energy and nutrition. Here are the key components that contribute to milk's status as a complete food:

Carbohydrates: Milk contains lactose, a natural sugar composed of glucose and galactose. Lactose serves as an energy source and provides sweetness to milk. It also aids in the absorption of calcium.

Proteins: Milk is a source of high-quality protein. The two primary types of proteins in milk are casein and whey. These proteins provide all essential amino acids needed for growth, repair, and overall body function. Casein makes up the majority of milk protein and has a slow-digesting nature, while whey is a rapidly digesting protein.

Fats: Milk contains a mix of saturated and unsaturated fats. It provides essential fatty acids and serves as a source of energy. The fat in milk is also essential for the absorption of fat-soluble vitamins like vitamin A, vitamin D, and vitamin K.

Vitamins: Milk is a rich source of various vitamins, including vitamin A, vitamin D, vitamin B12, and riboflavin (vitamin B2). These vitamins play essential roles in maintaining overall health. For example, vitamin D is necessary for calcium absorption and bone health, while vitamin A supports vision and immune function.

Minerals: Calcium is a standout mineral in milk, contributing to bone and teeth health, muscle function, and nerve signaling. Milk also contains significant amounts of phosphorus, potassium, and magnesium, which are essential for various bodily functions.

Water: Milk is primarily composed of water, which is vital for overall hydration and body functions.

Immune Factors: Milk contains immunoglobulins and other immune-enhancing components that provide immune system support, especially in newborns.

Growth Factors: Growth factors found in milk play a crucial role in promoting growth and development, particularly in infants.

B Vitamins: In addition to riboflavin (B2) and vitamin B12, milk provides other B vitamins like niacin (B3), pantothenic acid (B5), and pyridoxine (B6), which are important for energy metabolism.

Milk's nutrient density and balance make it an ideal food for promoting overall health and well-being. It is particularly important in the diets of children, adolescents, and the elderly. While milk is an excellent source of nutrition, individuals with lactose intolerance or dairy allergies should seek alternative sources of these nutrients. Additionally, sustainable and responsible milk production practices contribute to the environmental and ethical aspects of milk as a complete food.

The Power of Protein

Proteins are the building blocks of life, and milk is renowned for its protein content. Readers will gain insight into the various proteins found in milk, such as casein and whey, and how they contribute to muscle growth, tissue repair, and overall health.

Proteins are vital macronutrients with a wide range of functions in the body. They are often called the "building blocks of life" because they play essential roles in growth, repair, and maintenance of tissues and organs. Here's a look at the power of proteins:

1. Building and Repair: Proteins are crucial for the growth and repair of tissues. They provide the

amino acids necessary for the construction of new cells, such as muscle tissue, skin, and organs. This is particularly important in children, adolescents, and athletes who need protein for growth and recovery.

2. Enzymes: Enzymes are specialized proteins that catalyze biochemical reactions in the body. Without enzymes, many essential reactions would occur too slowly to sustain life. Enzymes are involved in processes such as digestion, metabolism, and detoxification.

3. Immune Function: Antibodies, which are part of the immune system, are proteins that help the body recognize and fight off pathogens like viruses and bacteria. A strong immune system depends on an adequate intake of protein.

4. Hormones: Several hormones, including insulin, growth hormone, and thyroid hormones, are proteins. These hormones regulate a wide range of physiological processes, from blood sugar control to growth and development.

5. Transport: Some proteins serve as carriers, transporting molecules such as oxygen (hemoglobin in red blood cells) and lipids (lipoproteins) throughout the body.

6. Structural Support: Structural proteins like collagen provide strength and support to tissues such as skin, tendons, and bones. Collagen, for example, is a major component of connective tissue.

7. Energy Source: While carbohydrates and fats are the body's primary energy sources, in the absence of sufficient carbohydrates and fats, proteins can be broken down and converted into energy.

8. Muscle Function: Muscle fibers are composed primarily of protein. Consuming adequate protein is crucial for maintaining and building muscle mass. Athletes and individuals engaging in resistance training often require higher protein intake to support muscle growth and recovery.

9. Satiety: Protein-rich foods tend to be more filling and can help control appetite. Including protein in your meals can aid in weight management by reducing overall calorie intake.

10. Amino Acids: Proteins are composed of amino acids, which are the basic building blocks of protein molecules. There are 20 different amino acids, and they can be combined in various ways to create a wide array of proteins with different structures and functions.

Sources of Protein: Dietary sources of protein include meat, poultry, fish, dairy products, eggs, legumes (beans, lentils, chickpeas), nuts, and seeds. Plant-based sources of protein can be particularly important for vegetarians and vegans.

Protein Requirements: Protein requirements vary depending on factors such as age, sex, activity level, and overall health. The Recommended Dietary Allowance (RDA) for protein for adults is approximately 0.8 grams of protein per kilogram of body weight per day. However, individuals with higher protein needs, such as athletes, pregnant and breastfeeding women, and people recovering from illness or injury, should adjust their intake accordingly.

Balanced Diet: A balanced diet includes a variety of protein sources to ensure a wide range of amino acids and other essential nutrients. A balanced diet also incorporates other macronutrients (carbohydrates and fats) and micronutrients (vitamins and minerals) for overall health.

Calcium: The Bone Builder

The role of calcium in milk is vital for bone health, and this section will emphasize how it supports the growth and maintenance of strong bones and teeth.

Readers will understand the importance of adequate calcium intake throughout life.

Vitamin D: The Sunshine Vitamin

Vitamin D is essential for calcium absorption and bone health. The chapter will explore the significance of vitamin D in milk, its role in preventing rickets, and its potential benefits for overall well-being.

The Nutritional Benefits of Dairy Fat

The chapter will explore the nutritional benefits of dairy fat and clarify the role of saturated fats in milk. Readers will understand the differences between full-fat, low-fat, and non-fat dairy products and how they fit into a balanced diet.

Dairy fat, often found in products like whole milk, butter, and cheese, has several nutritional benefits when consumed in moderation. Here are some of the advantages of including dairy fat in your diet:

Nutrient Absorption: Dietary fat is essential for the absorption of fat-soluble vitamins, including vitamins A, D, E, and K. Consuming dairy fat with foods rich in these vitamins can enhance their absorption and support overall health.

Satiety: Fats provide a feeling of fullness and satisfaction after meals. Including dairy fat in your diet can help control hunger and reduce overall calorie intake, potentially aiding in weight management.

Energy Source: Fat is a concentrated source of energy, providing 9 calories per gram. Dairy fat can be particularly beneficial for individuals with high energy demands, such as athletes and those engaged in physically demanding work.

Flavor and Palatability: Fats enhance the flavor and texture of foods. Dairy fat contributes to the rich and creamy textures of dairy products, making them more enjoyable and palatable.

Fatty Acids: Dairy fat contains a mix of fatty acids, including saturated and unsaturated fats. Some dairy fats are a source of healthy monounsaturated and polyunsaturated fats, which can have positive effects on heart health when consumed as part of a balanced diet.

Conjugated Linoleic Acid (CLA): Dairy fat, particularly from pasture-raised cows, can be a source of conjugated linoleic acid (CLA), which is associated with potential health benefits such as improved body composition and reduced inflammation.

Vitamin K2: Dairy fat can be a source of vitamin K2, which plays a role in bone health and may contribute to cardiovascular health.

Butyric Acid: Butter, in particular, contains butyric acid, which has been associated with potential anti-inflammatory and gut health benefits.

It's important to note that while dairy fat can offer nutritional benefits, it should be consumed in moderation as part of a balanced diet. Excessive consumption of saturated fats, including those found in dairy products, can increase the risk of heart disease. Therefore, it's advisable to choose low-fat or reduced-fat dairy options when possible, especially if you have specific dietary concerns or conditions.

Lactose: The Milk Sugar

Lactose, the natural sugar in milk, will be discussed in detail. Readers will learn about lactose intolerance, its symptoms, and how individuals with lactose intolerance can still enjoy dairy products with the help of lactase supplements and lactose-free alternatives.

Lactose is a natural sugar found in milk and dairy products. It plays a crucial role in milk's nutritional profile and taste. Here are key points about lactose:

1. Composition and Structure: Lactose is a disaccharide sugar composed of two simple sugar molecules, glucose and galactose, linked together. Its chemical structure is $C12H22O11$.

2. Primary Sugar in Milk: Lactose is the primary carbohydrate in milk, representing approximately 4.8-5.2% of the composition of cow's milk. The lactose content in milk may vary slightly among different animal species.

3. Natural Sweetness: Lactose is less sweet than other sugars like sucrose (table sugar). It provides a mild sweetness to milk and dairy products without being overly sugary.

4. Unique Digestion: Lactose requires a specific enzyme, lactase, for digestion. Lactase is produced in the small intestine and breaks down lactose into its component sugars, glucose, and galactose, which can then be absorbed into the bloodstream.

5. Lactose Intolerance: Some individuals, known as lactose-intolerant individuals, have insufficient levels of lactase, leading to difficulty in digesting lactose. This can result in symptoms such as

bloating, gas, and diarrhea after consuming dairy products.

6. Lactase Persistence: The ability to digest lactose is not universal among adults. However, some populations, particularly those with a history of dairy farming, have developed lactase persistence, allowing them to continue digesting lactose throughout adulthood.

7. Lactose-Free Dairy Products: To accommodate individuals with lactose intolerance, there are lactose-free dairy products available in the market. These products have been treated to break down lactose, making them easier to digest.

8. Nutritional Value: Lactose contributes calories to the diet, providing about 4 calories per gram. It also contributes carbohydrates, serving as an energy source.

9. Prebiotic Effects: Lactose may have prebiotic effects, promoting the growth of beneficial gut bacteria, particularly in individuals who can digest it.

10. Fermentation: Lactose can undergo fermentation by bacteria in dairy processes, leading to the production of products like yogurt and kefir. Fermentation converts lactose into lactic acid,

which contributes to the unique taste and texture of these dairy products.

Lactose is an integral part of milk's composition and plays a significant role in its nutritional value. While some individuals may experience lactose intolerance, which can limit their consumption of dairy products, there are options available to enjoy dairy without the discomfort associated with lactose intolerance, such as lactase supplements and lactose-free products. Additionally, dairy products offer a range of essential nutrients beyond lactose, including proteins, vitamins, and minerals.

Dairy in Different Stages of Life

The section will highlight the role of dairy in different stages of life, from infancy to old age. Readers will gain an understanding of how milk and dairy products support growth, development, and health throughout the lifespan.

"Dairy in Different Stages of Life" is an essential topic that highlights how milk and dairy products play a significant role in supporting growth, development, and overall health at various stages of life. Here's an overview of the role of dairy in different life stages:

Infancy and Early Childhood:

Breast Milk or Formula: In the early stages of life, infants rely on breast milk or infant formula as their primary source of nutrition. Breast milk is considered the gold standard, providing all essential nutrients, including proteins, fats, carbohydrates, vitamins, and minerals.

Transition to Dairy: As infants grow, they gradually transition to a diet that includes solid foods and dairy products. Dairy, such as whole milk and yogurt, is introduced to provide additional nutrients, particularly calcium and vitamin D, which are vital for bone and dental development.

Childhood and Adolescence:

Growth and Development: During childhood and adolescence, the body experiences rapid growth and development. Dairy products, including milk, cheese, and yogurt, are rich sources of high-quality proteins and calcium, which are essential for bone health, muscle growth, and overall development.

Nutrient-Rich Snacks: Dairy products can be incorporated into snacks and meals to ensure an adequate intake of essential nutrients like protein, calcium, and vitamins. These nutrients are critical for maintaining optimal health and supporting a healthy body weight.

Adulthood:

Bone Health: Dairy products continue to be important for maintaining bone density and preventing conditions like osteoporosis. They provide a readily absorbed source of calcium, which is essential for bone health throughout life.

Protein Intake: Dairy is an excellent source of high-quality protein, which is essential for muscle maintenance, immune function, and overall health. Consuming dairy products can help meet daily protein requirements.

Pregnancy and Lactation:

Nutrient Needs: During pregnancy and lactation, a woman's nutrient needs increase significantly. Dairy products can help provide essential nutrients like calcium, vitamin D, and protein, which are important for the health of both the mother and the developing fetus or infant.

Old Age:

Bone Health and Osteoporosis Prevention: In later stages of life, dairy products are crucial for maintaining bone health and preventing osteoporosis, a condition characterized by weakened bones. Calcium and vitamin D from dairy can help reduce the risk of fractures and bone-related diseases.

Protein for Muscle Health: As individuals age, muscle mass tends to decline. Consuming dairy products, which are rich in protein, can support muscle health and reduce the risk of sarcopenia, a condition characterized by muscle loss.

Digestibility: For some older individuals, dairy products may be easier to digest compared to certain other protein sources, making them a valuable addition to the diet.

It's important to note that while dairy products offer many nutritional benefits, some individuals may have lactose intolerance or dairy allergies, which can limit their consumption of dairy. In such cases, lactose-free dairy alternatives or other calcium-rich foods should be considered.

The role of dairy in different stages of life underscores its significance in providing essential nutrients for growth, development, and overall health, from infancy to old age. However, individual dietary needs may vary, and alternative sources of key nutrients should be explored for those with specific dietary restrictions or preferences.

Dairy and Healthy Eating Patterns

The chapter will explore how milk and dairy products fit into various healthy eating patterns, from Mediterranean to vegetarian diets. Readers will learn how to incorporate dairy into balanced meals for optimal nutrition.

"Dairy and Healthy Eating Patterns" is an important topic that emphasizes how milk and dairy products can be integrated into a variety of healthy eating patterns to promote optimal nutrition. Here's an overview of how dairy fits into different healthy dietary patterns:

1. Mediterranean Diet:

Yogurt and Cheese: In the Mediterranean diet, yogurt and cheese are commonly included. Yogurt can be consumed as a snack or part of a meal, while cheese is often used as a flavor-enhancing ingredient in salads, pasta, and sandwiches.

Olive Oil and Dairy: Olive oil and dairy complement each other in Mediterranean cuisine. Feta cheese and Greek yogurt are popular dairy choices, and they pair well with olive oil in dishes like Greek salads and tzatziki.

2. Vegetarian and Plant-Based Diets:

Dairy Alternatives: Many individuals following vegetarian and plant-based diets use dairy alternatives like almond milk, soy milk, and coconut yogurt to replace traditional dairy products.

Calcium and Protein: These diets often require careful planning to ensure adequate intake of calcium and protein, which can be sourced from fortified plant-based dairy alternatives.

3. DASH (Dietary Approaches to Stop Hypertension) Diet:

Low-Fat Dairy: The DASH diet emphasizes low-fat dairy products as part of a heart-healthy eating plan. Low-fat or fat-free milk, yogurt, and cheese are recommended to reduce saturated fat intake and support blood pressure management.

4. Balanced Diet:

Protein and Calcium: In a balanced diet, dairy products can contribute to the intake of essential nutrients, including high-quality protein and calcium. For example, milk can be consumed as a source of protein, and yogurt can provide probiotics and additional protein.

Desserts and Snacks: Dairy can be incorporated into desserts and snacks, such as parfaits, smoothies, and cheese platters, to make them more nutritious and satisfying.

5. Flexitarian Diet:

Variety of Options: The flexitarian diet allows for flexibility in dietary choices. Individuals can include dairy products or dairy alternatives based on their preferences and nutritional goals. Dairy provides protein and other nutrients that can complement a flexitarian diet.

6. Weight Management:

Satiety: Including dairy in meals and snacks can enhance satiety and help manage appetite, making it a valuable component of a weight management plan.

High-Protein Dairy: High-protein dairy products, such as Greek yogurt, can be particularly useful for those aiming to increase protein intake while controlling calorie consumption.

7. Child and Adolescent Nutrition:

Growth and Development: Milk and dairy products play a vital role in the nutrition of children and adolescents. These dairy products provide essential nutrients like calcium, vitamin D, and protein, which are crucial for growth and development.

It's important to note that the type of dairy and the amount consumed can vary depending on individual dietary preferences, nutritional needs, and health goals. Additionally, some individuals may have dietary restrictions or allergies that necessitate the use of dairy alternatives. Flexibility in incorporating dairy or dairy alternatives into a well-rounded diet allows individuals to optimize their nutrient intake while adhering to their specific dietary patterns.

The Role of Milk in Preventive Nutrition

This section will discuss the preventive aspects of milk and dairy consumption. Readers will gain insight into how dairy can play a role in preventing various health conditions, including osteoporosis, hypertension, and certain types of cancer.

"The Role of Milk in Preventive Nutrition" is an important topic that highlights how dairy consumption can contribute to the prevention of various health conditions. Here's an overview of the preventive aspects of milk and dairy consumption:

1. Osteoporosis Prevention:

Calcium: Milk and dairy products are rich sources of calcium, a mineral crucial for building and maintaining strong bones. Consuming an adequate amount of calcium throughout life, starting in childhood and continuing into adulthood, can help reduce the risk of osteoporosis, a condition characterized by weak and brittle bones.

2. Hypertension (High Blood Pressure) Management:

Calcium and Potassium: Dairy products provide essential nutrients like calcium and potassium, both of which are associated with blood pressure regulation. Adequate intake of these nutrients can help prevent and manage hypertension, reducing the risk of heart disease and stroke.

3. Colorectal Cancer Prevention:

Calcium: There is evidence to suggest that a higher intake of dietary calcium may be associated with a reduced risk of colorectal cancer. Dairy products are a major dietary source of calcium, and their consumption may contribute to this preventive effect.

4. Weight Management:

Satiety: Dairy products, particularly those rich in protein like Greek yogurt, can help enhance feelings of fullness and satiety. This can aid in weight management by reducing overall calorie intake and supporting a healthy body weight.

5. Dental Health:

Calcium and Phosphorus: Dairy products contain calcium and phosphorus, which are essential for strong teeth. Calcium plays a role in the formation of tooth enamel, while phosphorus helps maintain overall oral health.

6. Bone Health in Children and Adolescents:

Growth and Development: During childhood and adolescence, when bones are growing rapidly, consuming adequate calcium and vitamin D from dairy products is vital for achieving peak bone mass. This can reduce the risk of osteoporosis in later life.

7. Preeclampsia Prevention:

Calcium and Vitamin D: Adequate intake of calcium and vitamin D, which are found in dairy products, may play a role in reducing the risk of preeclampsia, a potentially serious pregnancy complication characterized by high blood pressure.

8. Metabolic Health:

Dairy Proteins: The proteins in dairy products can have beneficial effects on metabolic health. For example, some dairy proteins, like whey, have been linked to improved insulin sensitivity and glycemic control.

9. Mental Health:

Vitamin B12 and Vitamin D: Dairy products are sources of essential nutrients, including vitamin B12 and vitamin D, which are associated with mental health and mood regulation. Adequate intake of these nutrients can support overall well-being.

It's important to note that while milk and dairy consumption can play a role in preventive nutrition, dietary choices should be part of a comprehensive approach to health. A balanced diet that includes a variety of foods, along with other healthy lifestyle practices such as regular physical activity and not smoking, can significantly contribute to overall health and disease prevention. Individual dietary needs and preferences should also be taken into account when planning a preventive nutrition strategy.

The Future of Dairy Nutrition

The chapter will conclude by looking at the future of dairy nutrition, including the potential for fortified dairy products and innovations in dairy-based functional foods to meet specific nutritional needs and dietary preferences.

"The Future of Dairy Nutrition" is an exciting and dynamic topic that explores the evolving landscape of dairy nutrition. Here's an overview of what the future may hold for dairy nutrition:

1. Fortified Dairy Products:

Enhanced Nutrient Content: The future of dairy nutrition may see the development of more fortified dairy products. These products could be enriched with additional nutrients, such as vitamin D, omega-3 fatty acids, and probiotics, to meet specific dietary needs and address nutritional deficiencies.

2. Personalized Nutrition:

Tailored Dairy Solutions: With advances in personalized nutrition, dairy products could be customized to individual dietary requirements. For example, personalized dairy products might provide targeted nutrients based on an individual's genetic makeup, health goals, and nutritional needs.

3. Dairy-Based Functional Foods:

Innovative Functional Ingredients: Dairy-based functional foods may become increasingly popular. These foods can include probiotic yogurt for gut health, fortified milk for bone health, and dairy protein shakes for muscle recovery. The innovation in functional ingredients will cater to specific health and wellness trends.

4. Sustainable Dairy Nutrition:

Environmental Considerations: The future of dairy nutrition will likely place a stronger emphasis on sustainability. This may involve developing more sustainable dairy farming practices, reducing the carbon footprint of dairy products, and exploring alternative protein sources with lower environmental impacts.

5. Non-Dairy Alternatives:

Plant-Based Dairy Alternatives: As plant-based milk and dairy alternatives continue to gain popularity, the future of dairy nutrition may involve a broader range of non-dairy alternatives like almond milk, soy yogurt, and cashew-based cheese.

6. Dairy and Technology:

Digital Tools: Technology will play a role in dairy nutrition with the development of digital tools and apps that help consumers make informed choices about their dairy consumption based on their health goals, dietary preferences, and nutritional needs.

7. Dairy in Global Nutrition:

Global Reach: Dairy nutrition will continue to evolve as it reaches more regions and populations worldwide. Innovations in dairy products and their adaptation to local preferences and nutritional requirements will be a key aspect of the future.

8. Research and Discoveries:

Ongoing Studies: Ongoing research will uncover new health benefits and nutritional properties of dairy products. These discoveries may lead to the development of novel dairy-based products that promote health and well-being.

9. Regulatory Frameworks:

Guidelines and Labeling: Regulatory frameworks for dairy nutrition will evolve, with clearer guidelines on product labeling, health claims, and quality standards. This will ensure consumers have accurate and transparent information about the nutritional content of dairy products.

10. Nutritional Education: - Consumer Awareness: Nutritional education will continue to be a key factor in shaping the future of dairy nutrition. Increased awareness and understanding of the health benefits of dairy will influence consumer choices and dietary preferences.

The future of dairy nutrition is marked by innovation, adaptability, and a commitment to meeting the diverse and evolving nutritional needs of consumers. It will involve a blend of tradition and modernity, with a focus on providing delicious and nutrient-rich dairy products that support overall health and well-being. As the field of nutrition advances, so too will the opportunities to enjoy dairy as a versatile and essential component of a balanced diet.

The Versatility of Dairy Nutrition

The chapter will continue by exploring the versatility of dairy nutrition in various dietary patterns and cuisines. Readers will learn how milk and dairy products have adapted to different cultural and culinary traditions, providing essential nutrients while adding richness and flavor to a wide range of dishes.

"The Versatility of Dairy Nutrition" is a fascinating exploration of how milk and dairy products have adapted to various dietary patterns and cuisines around the world. Here's an overview of the versatility of dairy nutrition in different cultures and culinary traditions:

1. Mediterranean Cuisine:

Greek Yogurt: Greek yogurt is a staple in Mediterranean cuisine, used in dishes like tzatziki, a yogurt and cucumber sauce, and as a creamy dessert with honey and fruits.

2. Indian Cuisine:

Paneer: Paneer is a fresh Indian cheese commonly used in vegetarian dishes, providing a rich source of protein. It's featured in dishes like saag paneer and paneer tikka.

3. Middle Eastern Cuisine:

Labneh: Labneh, a strained yogurt cheese, is a key component in Middle Eastern cuisine. It's used in savory and sweet dishes, such as dips, salads, and desserts.

4. Italian Cuisine:

Cheeses: Italian cuisine features a variety of dairy products, including Parmesan, mozzarella, ricotta, and gorgonzola. These cheeses are used in pasta dishes, pizzas, and desserts like tiramisu.

5. Mexican Cuisine:

Queso Fresco: Queso fresco, a fresh cheese, is often used in Mexican cuisine, adding a creamy element to tacos, salads, and enchiladas.

6. Asian Cuisine:

Coconut Milk: In Asian cuisine, coconut milk is a common dairy alternative used in curries, soups, and desserts. It provides a creamy and nutty flavor.

7. French Cuisine:

Cream and Butter: French cuisine is renowned for its use of dairy, including cream and butter in sauces, pastries, and decadent desserts like crème brûlée.

8. Eastern European Cuisine:

Sour Cream: Eastern European cuisine incorporates sour cream in dishes like borscht, pierogi, and stroganoff. It adds a tangy and creamy element.

9. African Cuisine:

Fulbe Yogurt: In African countries like Senegal, Fulbe yogurt is a traditional fermented yogurt used in both savory and sweet dishes.

10. Global Fusion Cuisine: - Cross-Cultural Blending: Fusion cuisine often combines dairy ingredients from different cultural traditions. Examples include Mexican-inspired lasagna with crema and Indian-inspired mango lassi with yogurt.

11. Vegetarian and Vegan Cuisine: - Dairy Alternatives: Vegetarian and vegan cuisines incorporate dairy alternatives like almond milk, coconut yogurt, and cashew-based cheese into recipes.

12. Nutrient-Rich Additions: - Protein and Calcium: Dairy products provide essential nutrients such as high-quality protein and calcium, enhancing the nutritional value of various dishes.

13. Taste and Texture Enhancement: - Flavor and Creaminess: Dairy products contribute to the flavor and texture of dishes, enhancing the overall dining experience.

14. Culinary Adaptations: - Cultural Fusion: As cuisines and cultures intersect, culinary adaptations occur, creating unique dishes that incorporate dairy in innovative ways.

The versatility of dairy nutrition is evident in its ability to enhance a wide range of global cuisines, from traditional recipes passed down through generations to contemporary fusion creations. Dairy products bring not only essential nutrients but also a world of flavor and texture to dishes, making them a cherished and adaptable part of culinary traditions around the globe.

Dairy Nutrition and Dietary Guidelines

Readers will gain insight into how dietary guidelines around the world emphasize the importance of dairy consumption for a balanced and nutritious diet. This section will explore recommended daily servings and the various dairy products that contribute to meeting these guidelines.

"Dairy Nutrition and Dietary Guidelines" is a significant topic that sheds light on how dietary guidelines worldwide emphasize the role of dairy consumption in maintaining a balanced and nutritious diet. Here's an overview of how dietary guidelines recommend daily servings and the diverse dairy products that contribute to fulfilling these guidelines:

1. United States:

Dietary Guidelines for Americans: In the United States, the Dietary Guidelines for Americans recommend daily dairy consumption. The guidelines suggest consuming three servings of dairy per day, which can include milk, yogurt, cheese, and fortified dairy alternatives.

2. Canada:

Canada's Food Guide: Canada's Food Guide encourages individuals to consume a variety of dairy products daily. This includes milk, yogurt, and cheese, with an emphasis on choosing lower-fat options.

3. United Kingdom:

Eatwell Guide: The United Kingdom's Eatwell Guide suggests including dairy or dairy alternatives in daily meals and snacks. It recommends choosing lower-fat and lower-sugar options.

4. Australia:

Australian Dietary Guidelines: The Australian Dietary Guidelines advise consuming dairy or dairy alternatives daily for the intake of calcium and other nutrients. The guidelines recommend choosing mostly reduced-fat options.

5. European Union:

European Dietary Guidelines: Dietary guidelines in the European Union typically promote the inclusion of dairy products in daily meals. These guidelines recommend a variety of dairy options, including yogurt and cheese, as part of a balanced diet.

6. India:

Indian Dietary Guidelines: In India, dietary guidelines recommend the consumption of milk and milk products as part of a balanced diet. These products include milk, yogurt, and traditional dairy items like paneer.

7. China:

Chinese Dietary Guidelines: China's dietary guidelines emphasize the consumption of dairy products, particularly milk, to meet calcium and protein needs. Dairy alternatives like soy milk are also considered.

8. Global Nutrition Recommendations:

World Health Organization (WHO): The World Health Organization acknowledges the importance of dairy products in meeting nutritional needs. Dairy is especially emphasized for children and adolescents to support growth and development.

9. Special Populations:

Pregnancy and Lactation: Dietary guidelines often highlight the significance of dairy for pregnant and lactating women due to increased calcium requirements.

Infants and Young Children: For infants, breastfeeding is recommended, but for young children, guidelines may include age-appropriate dairy foods.

10. Dairy Alternatives: Dietary guidelines increasingly accommodate dairy alternatives for individuals with lactose intolerance or those following vegetarian or vegan diets. These guidelines emphasize the importance of choosing fortified alternatives to ensure adequate nutrient intake.

11. Quality and Quantity: Guidelines typically stress the importance of choosing high-quality, nutrient-dense dairy products and consuming them in appropriate quantities to meet daily nutrient needs without excessive calorie intake.

Dietary guidelines play a vital role in guiding individuals toward a balanced and nutritious diet. The inclusion of dairy products in these guidelines underscores their value as a source of essential nutrients, such as calcium, vitamin D, protein, and more. It also acknowledges the adaptability of dairy nutrition to various dietary patterns and preferences, providing a valuable source of nutrients for diverse populations.

Dairy and Bone Health

The role of dairy nutrition in bone health will be a central focus. Readers will understand the critical connection between calcium and vitamin D in dairy products and their role in building and maintaining strong bones and preventing conditions like osteoporosis.

"Dairy and Bone Health" is a critical topic that highlights the essential role of dairy nutrition in supporting bone health. Here's an overview of the central connection between calcium, vitamin D, and their role in building and maintaining strong bones:

1. Calcium for Bone Health:

Bone Mineralization: Calcium is a fundamental mineral that plays a crucial role in bone health. It is a key component of bone mineralization, the process by which minerals are deposited into the bone matrix, making bones strong and dense.

Peak Bone Mass: Adequate calcium intake during childhood and adolescence is essential for achieving peak bone mass, which is the maximum bone density attained during a person's lifetime. This is a critical factor in reducing the risk of osteoporosis later in life.

Osteoporosis Prevention: Insufficient calcium intake can lead to reduced bone density, increasing the risk of osteoporosis, a condition characterized by fragile and brittle bones.

2. Vitamin D for Calcium Absorption:

Calcium Absorption: Vitamin D is necessary for the absorption of calcium from the intestines into the bloodstream. Without sufficient vitamin D, the body cannot effectively utilize the calcium consumed through diet or supplements.

Sunlight and Vitamin D: The body can produce vitamin D when exposed to sunlight. However, dietary sources of vitamin D, including fortified dairy products, are vital, especially in regions with limited sun exposure.

3. Role of Dairy in Bone Health:

High-Quality Calcium: Dairy products are among the best dietary sources of calcium. They provide highly bioavailable and easily absorbable calcium, making them an effective way to support bone health.

Additional Nutrients: Dairy products offer additional nutrients important for bone health, such as protein, phosphorus, and magnesium.

Yogurt and Fermented Dairy: Yogurt and some fermented dairy products may contain probiotics that could contribute to gut health and overall well-being.

4. Age and Bone Health:

Lifelong Importance: Maintaining strong bones is a lifelong endeavor. Adequate calcium and vitamin D intake are important throughout all life stages, from childhood and adolescence to adulthood and into the senior years.

Senior Health: In older adults, especially post-menopausal women, the risk of bone loss and fractures increases. Adequate dairy consumption can help mitigate this risk.

5. Dietary Considerations:

Dietary Preferences: For those who are lactose intolerant or have dairy allergies, there are lactose-free and dairy-free options and fortified dairy alternatives available to meet calcium and vitamin D needs.

Balanced Diet: While dairy is a valuable source of bone-boosting nutrients, it's important to consume a balanced diet that includes a variety of other foods rich in calcium and vitamin D, such as leafy greens, fortified cereals, and fatty fish.

The role of dairy in bone health is pivotal, with calcium and vitamin D being central components of strong and healthy bones. Dairy products, including milk, yogurt, and cheese, provide a convenient and effective way to ensure adequate calcium and vitamin D intake, ultimately contributing to the prevention of osteoporosis and the maintenance of skeletal health throughout life.

Dairy and Cardiovascular Health

The chapter will explore the impact of dairy nutrition on cardiovascular health. Readers will gain an understanding of the relationship between dairy fats and heart health, as well as the potential benefits of consuming low-fat and non-fat dairy products.

The relationship between dairy nutrition and cardiovascular health is a crucial aspect of overall well-being. Readers will gain insight into the impact of dairy products on heart health, exploring the roles of various dairy components and their potential effects on cardiovascular risk factors.

1. Dairy Fats and Heart Health:

Saturated Fats: Some dairy products, such as whole milk and butter, contain saturated fats, which were traditionally associated with increased cardiovascular risk. However, recent research suggests that the relationship between saturated fats and heart health is more nuanced than once believed.

Dietary Guidelines: Many dietary guidelines now recommend consuming lower-fat dairy options as part of a heart-healthy diet. This includes options like skim milk, low-fat yogurt, and reduced-fat cheese.

2. Unsaturated Fats in Dairy:

Monounsaturated and Polyunsaturated Fats: Some dairy products, particularly cheese, contain monounsaturated and polyunsaturated fats. These types of fats may have potential cardiovascular benefits, including improving cholesterol profiles.

3. Dairy Proteins and Blood Pressure:

Protein and Blood Pressure Regulation: Dairy proteins, including casein and whey, may play a role in regulating blood pressure. Some studies suggest that consuming dairy proteins can have a blood pressure-lowering effect.

4. Calcium and Blood Pressure:

Calcium's Role: Calcium, abundant in dairy products, may contribute to blood pressure regulation. Adequate calcium intake is associated with a reduced risk of hypertension, a major risk factor for cardiovascular disease.

5. Potassium and Magnesium:

Electrolytes in Dairy: Dairy products are sources of essential minerals like potassium and magnesium, which are important for heart health. These minerals play a role in maintaining healthy blood pressure and heart rhythm.

6. Probiotics and Gut Health:

Fermented Dairy Products: Some fermented dairy products, like yogurt, contain probiotics that can positively impact gut health. Emerging research suggests that a healthy gut microbiome may be linked to cardiovascular health.

7. Dairy and Lipid Profiles:

Cholesterol and Triglycerides: The influence of dairy products on lipid profiles (cholesterol and triglyceride levels) remains a topic of ongoing research. The relationship between dairy fats and lipids can vary among individuals.

8. Whole vs. Low-Fat Dairy:

Balancing Nutrients: The choice between whole and low-fat dairy depends on individual dietary needs and goals. Low-fat dairy is often recommended for those looking to manage their calorie and saturated fat intake.

9. Moderation and a Balanced Diet:

Context Matters: Cardiovascular health is influenced by an individual's overall dietary pattern. Including dairy as part of a balanced diet, alongside fruits, vegetables, whole grains, and lean proteins, is a holistic approach to supporting heart health.

10. Lactose-Free and Dairy Alternatives: - Diverse Options: For individuals with lactose intolerance or dairy allergies, lactose-free and dairy-free alternatives are available, providing options that support both dietary preferences and cardiovascular health.

Dairy and Weight Management

The section will delve into the role of dairy nutrition in weight management. Readers will explore how the protein and calcium in dairy products can support weight loss and maintenance, and how these products can be incorporated into a calorie-conscious diet.

The relationship between dairy nutrition and weight management is a topic of significant interest in the context of overall health and wellness. Readers will gain insight into how dairy products can play a role in weight management and understand the various mechanisms involved.

1. Protein and Satiety:

High-Quality Protein: Dairy products, such as milk, yogurt, and cheese, are rich sources of high-quality protein. Protein has a satiating effect, helping individuals feel fuller for longer, which can assist in controlling appetite and overall calorie intake.

2. Calcium and Fat Metabolism:

Calcium's Role: Calcium, abundant in dairy, may contribute to weight management by influencing fat metabolism. Adequate calcium intake is associated with reduced fat absorption in the intestines and increased fat breakdown.

3. Dairy Fats and Satiety:

Balancing Fats: The type of dairy fat can impact satiety. Consuming dairy products with healthy fats, such as monounsaturated and polyunsaturated fats, may be more satiating and supportive of weight management.

4. Probiotics and Gut Health:

Fermented Dairy Products: Some dairy products, like yogurt, contain probiotics that can positively influence gut health. Emerging research suggests that a healthy gut microbiome may be linked to weight management.

5. Portion Control:

Mindful Consumption: Dairy products can be calorie-dense, so portion control is important, especially for individuals aiming to manage their weight. Choosing lower-calorie dairy options can support weight goals.

6. Balanced Diet:**

Incorporating Variety: Including a variety of foods in a balanced diet is key to effective weight management. Dairy products can be part of a well-rounded meal plan that includes fruits, vegetables, whole grains, and lean proteins.

7. Dairy as a Protein Source:

Substituting for Other Proteins: For individuals aiming to manage their weight, dairy products can be used to replace less nutritious, higher-calorie protein sources, contributing to overall calorie reduction.

8. Physical Activity:

Complementing Exercise: Weight management is a holistic approach that includes not only dietary choices but also physical activity. Dairy products can be part of a diet supporting an active lifestyle.

9. Lactose-Free and Dairy Alternatives:

Diverse Options: For individuals with lactose intolerance or dairy allergies, lactose-free and dairy-free alternatives offer choices to support both dietary preferences and weight management goals.

10. Individual Variation: - Personalized Approach: Weight management is highly individual. What works for one person may not work for another. It's essential to find a dietary pattern that aligns with individual preferences and needs.

11. Behavioral Factors: - Mindful Eating: Weight management is influenced by not only what we eat but also how we eat. Mindful eating, which

involves being aware of hunger and fullness cues, can be a valuable strategy in combination with dairy consumption.

Dairy in Pediatric Nutrition

Readers will gain insight into the significance of dairy in pediatric nutrition. This section will discuss how milk and dairy products are essential for children's growth and development, providing the necessary nutrients for strong bones and overall health.

Dairy nutrition plays a critical role in pediatric nutrition, supporting the growth, development, and overall health of children. This section will explore the significance of dairy products in children's diets and the benefits they offer:

1. Growth and Development:

Calcium for Bone Growth: Dairy products are rich sources of calcium, which is essential for the development of strong and healthy bones in children. Adequate calcium intake is crucial during childhood and adolescence to achieve peak bone mass.

Protein for Muscle Development: Dairy provides high-quality protein necessary for muscle development and overall growth in children.

2. Nutrient Density:

Multiple Nutrients: Dairy products are nutrient-dense, offering a range of essential nutrients, including calcium, vitamin D, protein, and various vitamins and minerals.

Probiotics in Yogurt: Some dairy products, such as yogurt, contain probiotics that may promote gut health, which is linked to overall well-being.

3. Weight Management:

Satiety: Dairy's protein content can help children feel full and satisfied, potentially contributing to weight management by reducing the risk of excessive calorie consumption.

4. Lactose Intolerance and Alternatives:

Managing Lactose Intolerance: For children with lactose intolerance, lactose-free and dairy alternatives can provide essential nutrients without causing digestive discomfort.

5. Transitioning to Solid Foods:

Introducing Dairy: Dairy products, like plain yogurt or cheese, can be introduced as part of a child's transition to solid foods. These foods provide a range of nutrients, including protein and calcium, important for growth and development.

6. Variety in the Diet:

Balanced Diet: Including a variety of foods, including dairy, in a child's diet is important for balanced nutrition. This variety helps children get a wide range of essential nutrients.

7. Portion Control:

Appropriate Portions: Children have specific calorie and nutrient needs. Proper portion control ensures that they receive the necessary nutrients without excess calories.

8. Allergies and Dietary Preferences:

Managing Allergies: For children with dairy allergies, it's important to avoid dairy products and find suitable alternatives. Nutrient-fortified non-dairy milk alternatives can be considered.

Dietary Preferences: Some children may follow vegetarian or vegan diets. In such cases, it's essential to plan diets carefully to ensure adequate intake of calcium, protein, and other nutrients that dairy typically provides.

9. Promoting Healthy Habits:

Long-Term Benefits: Encouraging healthy eating habits in childhood can have long-term health benefits. Children who learn to enjoy dairy and other nutritious foods are more likely to maintain a balanced diet as they grow.

Lactose Intolerance and Alternatives

The section will address lactose intolerance, offering information on the condition, its prevalence, and strategies for managing it. Readers will learn about lactose-free dairy alternatives, lactase supplements, and the importance of meeting nutritional needs without dairy.

Lactose Intolerance:

Definition: Lactose intolerance is the inability to digest lactose, a natural sugar found in milk and dairy products, due to insufficient production of the enzyme lactase in the small intestine.

Symptoms: Common symptoms include bloating, gas, diarrhea, and stomach cramps after consuming lactose-containing foods or drinks.

Diagnosis: It is typically diagnosed through symptom assessment, hydrogen breath test, or a lactose tolerance test.

Management: Lactose-intolerant individuals can manage their condition by reducing or avoiding lactose-containing foods or using lactase supplements to aid digestion.

Lactose-Free Dairy Alternatives:

Lactose-Free Milk: Lactose-free milk is cow's milk with added lactase enzyme, which breaks down lactose into its digestible components, glucose, and galactose. This makes it suitable for lactose-intolerant individuals.

Lactose-Free Yogurt: Similar to lactose-free milk, lactose-free yogurt is made from cow's milk treated with lactase enzyme to eliminate lactose.

Lactose-Free Cheese: Some types of lactose-free cheese are available, typically made from lactose-free milk.

Dairy Alternatives:

Plant-Based Milk: A wide range of plant-based milk alternatives, such as almond, soy, oat, and coconut milk, are available. They are naturally lactose-free and can be used as substitutes for cow's milk in various applications.

Non-Dairy Yogurt: Plant-based yogurts made from almond, coconut, soy, or other alternatives provide options for those who cannot consume dairy.

Non-Dairy Cheese: Dairy-free cheese alternatives, often made from ingredients like nuts or soy, offer options for lactose-intolerant individuals who enjoy cheese flavors.

Lactose-Free Ice Cream: Lactose-free versions of ice cream are available in various flavors and are suitable for those with lactose intolerance.

Nutritional Considerations:

Fortified Varieties: Many dairy alternatives are fortified with calcium, vitamin D, and other nutrients to make them nutritionally comparable to dairy milk.

Protein Content: Check the protein content in non-dairy alternatives, as it can vary. Soy milk, for instance, tends to have a higher protein content than almond or rice milk.

Allergen Considerations: Some individuals with lactose intolerance may also have allergies to nuts, soy, or other ingredients commonly used in dairy alternatives, so it's essential to consider allergen information.

Cooking and Baking:

Substitution: Dairy alternatives can often be used as direct substitutes for dairy milk in cooking and baking. Be aware that flavors and textures may vary, so experimentation may be necessary.

Thickness and Texture: The consistency of non-dairy alternatives can vary. Choose the appropriate one for specific recipes, such as almond milk for a lighter texture or coconut milk for a creamier one.

Homemade Alternatives:

Nut Milk: Homemade nut milks, like almond or cashew milk, can be prepared by blending nuts with water and straining the mixture. This allows for customization of flavor and thickness.

Oat Milk: Oat milk can be made at home by blending oats with water and straining the mixture. It's a versatile option for various culinary applications.

Individual Preferences:

Taste Preferences: Taste and texture preferences vary widely. Some people prefer the taste of specific non-dairy alternatives over others, so it's a matter of personal preference.

Environmental and Ethical Factors: Some individuals choose non-dairy alternatives for environmental or ethical reasons, such as reducing the carbon footprint associated with dairy farming or avoiding animal products.

Lactose intolerance is a common condition, and there are various alternatives available to accommodate dietary preferences and restrictions. These alternatives can provide a similar taste and nutritional value to dairy products while catering to the specific needs of individuals with lactose intolerance or those who choose non-dairy options for various reasons.

Dairy Nutrition and Special Diets

Readers will explore the adaptation of dairy nutrition to special diets, including lactose-free, dairy-free, vegetarian, and vegan eating patterns. The section will highlight dairy alternatives and fortifications to meet specific dietary needs.

Dairy nutrition can be adapted to various special diets and dietary preferences. This section will explore how dairy fits into different dietary patterns and the considerations for specific dietary needs:

1. Vegetarian and Vegan Diets:

Vegetarian Diets: Vegetarians exclude meat but may include dairy and dairy products. They can incorporate dairy for essential nutrients such as calcium and protein.

Vegan Diets: Vegans exclude all animal products, including dairy. They can opt for plant-based milk alternatives fortified with calcium and vitamin D, as well as other non-dairy sources of calcium like fortified tofu, leafy greens, and almonds.

2. Gluten-Free Diets:

Celiac Disease: Individuals with celiac disease must avoid gluten-containing grains like wheat, barley, and rye. Most dairy products are naturally gluten-free, making them safe for those with celiac disease.

3. Paleo and Whole30 Diets:

Paleo Diet: The paleo diet excludes dairy, along with grains, legumes, and processed foods. Individuals following this diet rely on other sources of calcium and nutrients.

Whole30 Diet: The Whole30 diet eliminates dairy, grains, legumes, and added sugars for a month.

After the diet, individuals can reintroduce dairy to assess tolerance.

4. Low-Carb and Keto Diets:

Low-Carb Diet: Low-carb diets can include dairy products with lower carbohydrate content, like plain yogurt and hard cheeses. These can provide protein and healthy fats while keeping carbohydrate intake in check.

Keto Diet: The ketogenic diet emphasizes high fat intake, making full-fat dairy products like butter and heavy cream suitable for this diet. Dairy can provide a source of healthy fats and protein while minimizing carbohydrate consumption.

5. FODMAP Diet:

FODMAPs: The FODMAP diet is designed for individuals with irritable bowel syndrome (IBS) and involves reducing fermentable carbohydrates that can trigger symptoms. Some dairy products are low in FODMAPs, making them suitable for this diet.

6. Lactose Intolerance:

Lactase Supplements: Individuals with lactose intolerance can take lactase supplements to help digest lactose when consuming dairy.

Lactose-Free Products: Lactose-free dairy products are suitable alternatives for those with lactose intolerance.

7. Balanced Diets:

Overall Nutrient Balance: In all dietary patterns, it's essential to ensure a balance of nutrients, including calcium and protein. Individuals not consuming dairy should incorporate other sources of these nutrients, such as fortified foods, leafy greens, nuts, and legumes.

8. Cultural and Regional Diets:

Cultural Preferences: Diets vary significantly based on cultural and regional preferences. In some cultures, dairy is a staple, while in others, it is rarely consumed. Dietary choices should align with cultural and regional preferences.

9. Personalization:

Individual Needs: Dietary needs vary from person to person. It's important to customize one's diet based on individual preferences, health goals, and dietary restrictions.

Adapting dairy nutrition to special diets requires careful consideration of dietary preferences and health needs. There are often suitable alternatives that provide essential nutrients while aligning with specific dietary patterns. Individuals should consult with healthcare professionals or dietitians for personalized guidance on how to meet their nutritional requirements while adhering to their chosen diet.

CHAPTER SIX

Cheese: The Dairy World's Masterpiece

Cheese, with its countless varieties and complex flavors, stands as one of the most celebrated and diverse creations in the world of dairy. This chapter delves into the art and science of cheese production, the rich cultural significance of cheese, and its versatility in culinary traditions around the globe.

The Origin of Cheese

The chapter begins with a historical exploration of cheese, unraveling its mysterious origins and early adoption by various civilizations. Readers will learn how cheese-making techniques have evolved over centuries.

The origin of cheese is a fascinating journey that dates back thousands of years. Here's an overview of how cheese, one of the oldest and most beloved dairy products, came into existence:

1. Discovery of Cheese by Accident:

The exact origin of cheese is not documented, but it is believed to have been discovered by accident.

Legend has it that cheese was discovered when an enterprising traveler stored milk in a container made from an animal's stomach. The rennet enzymes in the stomach lining curdled the milk, resulting in the first cheese.

2. Early Beginnings in the Middle East:

Cheese production likely began in the Middle East, particularly in the regions of present-day Iran and Turkey.

Ancient texts from Mesopotamia (modern-day Iraq) dating back to around 2000 BC mention cheese production.

3. Spread Across Europe:

Cheese-making techniques were passed down through generations and spread to other regions.

Cheese production became a common practice in ancient Greece and Rome, with various types of cheese mentioned in historical texts.

4. Monasteries and Medieval Europe:

Monasteries played a significant role in the preservation and advancement of cheese-making knowledge during the Middle Ages in Europe.

Monks developed and recorded various cheese recipes, contributing to the diversity of cheese types.

5. European Cheese Traditions:

European countries developed their own unique cheese traditions, resulting in the creation of numerous varieties of cheese.

Cheese-making practices were influenced by factors such as local milk sources, climate, and regional preferences.

6. Colonial Influence:

European settlers brought cheese-making traditions to the Americas during the colonial period.

In the United States, cheese production became a significant industry in the 19th century.

7. Industrialization and Modern Cheese Production:

The industrial revolution in the 19th century brought advancements in cheese production technology.

Cheese production transitioned from small-scale artisanal practices to large-scale, industrial processes.

8. Global Popularity:

Today, cheese is enjoyed worldwide and is a staple in many cuisines.

Various countries have their own iconic cheese varieties, such as Cheddar in the United Kingdom, Brie in France, and Gouda in the Netherlands.

9. Cheese-Making Process:

The basic process of cheese making involves curdling milk, separating the curds from the whey, and aging the curds to develop the flavor and texture.

Different types of cheese are created by varying the source of milk (cow, goat, sheep), the bacteria or enzymes used, the aging process, and added flavorings (herbs, spices).

Cheese has a rich history and continues to be a versatile and beloved dairy product used in a wide range of culinary applications. Its diverse flavors, textures, and uses make it a central ingredient in countless dishes worldwide.

The Cheese-Making Process

The cheese-making process is a complex craft, and this section will break it down step by step. Readers will understand the fundamental stages, from coagulation and curd formation to the role of microbes and enzymes in cheese maturation.

The cheese-making process is a fascinating and intricate series of steps that transform milk into the wide array of cheese varieties we enjoy today. While there are numerous cheese types, the fundamental steps in cheese making remain relatively consistent. Here is an overview of the cheese-making process:

1. Milk Selection:

The process begins with selecting the type of milk used, which can come from cows, goats, sheep, or other mammals. The quality of the milk, including its fat content and freshness, plays a significant role in the final cheese's characteristics.

2. Coagulation:

Coagulation is the process of turning milk into curds and whey. This step involves adding a coagulant to the milk, traditionally rennet (an enzyme found in the stomach lining of animals) or acid (like lemon juice or vinegar).

The coagulant causes the milk to curdle, forming solid curds and liquid whey.

3. Curd Cutting:

Once the milk has coagulated, the curds are cut into small pieces to release more whey. The size of the curds and the cutting method can affect the cheese's final texture.

4. Whey Separation:

The curds and whey are then separated. This can be done by carefully pouring off the whey or by using tools like cheesecloth, a slotted spoon, or a cheese mold.

The remaining curds will form the foundation of the cheese.

5. Curd Cooking and Shaping:

The curds are gently heated and stirred. The temperature and cooking time vary depending on the type of cheese being made.

Curd shaping involves pressing the curds into molds or containers, which helps eliminate more whey and solidify the cheese.

6. Salting:

Salt is often added to the cheese curds for flavor and preservation. The type of salt, as well as the method of application, can vary.

7. Cheese Aging:

Cheese aging is a critical step in cheese making. The cheese is placed in a controlled environment to develop flavor and texture. Aging can last from a few weeks to several years, depending on the cheese type.

During aging, various biochemical changes occur, including the breakdown of proteins and fats, which contribute to the development of the cheese's unique characteristics.

8. Final Packaging:

After aging, the cheese is usually cut into appropriate portions, shaped, and packaged for sale and consumption.

The above steps are fundamental to the cheese-making process, but the specific details can vary significantly from one cheese type to another.

Factors such as the choice of milk, the use of specific bacteria or molds, the aging conditions, and any additional flavorings (such as herbs or spices) can result in a wide variety of cheeses, each with its own distinct taste, texture, and appearance.

Cheese makers worldwide have honed their craft over centuries, resulting in an incredible diversity of cheeses that delight palates around the globe.

Cheese Varieties: A World of Taste

Readers will embark on a global journey through the various cheese varieties. From soft and creamy Brie to pungent blue cheese and aged cheddar, this section will explore the diversity of flavors, textures, and forms that cheese can take.

Cheese varieties span the globe, offering an extensive range of tastes, textures, and culinary possibilities. Here is a selection of cheese varieties from around the world, each with its unique characteristics and regional influences:

1. Cheddar (United Kingdom):

Taste and Texture: Cheddar is known for its rich, creamy texture and a flavor that ranges from mild to sharp, depending on aging.

Uses: It’s a versatile cheese used in sandwiches, salads, or melted in various dishes.

2. Brie (France):

Taste and Texture: Brie is soft and creamy with a mild, earthy flavor and a white, edible rind.

Uses: It’s often served as a dessert cheese or in baked dishes.

3. Gouda (Netherlands):

Taste and Texture: Gouda is a mild, semi-hard cheese with a slightly sweet, nutty flavor.

Uses: It’s perfect for snacking, melting, or slicing in sandwiches.

4. Parmigiano-Reggiano (Italy):

Taste and Texture: Parmigiano-Reggiano, known as the "King of Cheese," is hard, grainy, and has a salty, nutty flavor.

Uses: It’s grated on pasta, risotto, and salads and is often served with balsamic vinegar.

5. Manchego (Spain):

Taste and Texture: Manchego is a semi-firm, sheep’s milk cheese with a nutty, slightly tangy taste.

Uses: It’s great for snacking, serving with olives, or grating over dishes.

6. Roquefort (France):

Taste and Texture: Roquefort is a blue cheese with a creamy texture and a strong, tangy flavor.

Uses: It’s excellent for dressings, spreads, or enjoying on a cheese platter.

7. Swiss (Switzerland):

Taste and Texture: Swiss cheese has a mild, slightly nutty taste and is characterized by its holes or "eyes."

Uses: It’s famous for melting in fondues and sandwiches.

8. Feta (Greece):

Taste and Texture: Feta is a crumbly, tangy cheese with a salty flavor.

Uses: It’s ideal for Greek salads, pastries, or as a table cheese.

9. Mozzarella (Italy):

Taste and Texture: Mozzarella is a soft, mild cheese with a fresh, milky flavor.

Uses: It’s the classic choice for pizza, caprese salads, and lasagna.

10. Paneer (India):

Taste and Texture: Paneer is a fresh, non-melting cheese with a mild, milky flavor.

Uses: It’s widely used in Indian cuisine, particularly in dishes like palak paneer and paneer tikka.

11. Queso Fresco (Latin America):

Taste and Texture: Queso fresco is a fresh, crumbly cheese with a slightly salty, mild flavor.

Uses: It’s popular in Mexican, Central, and South American cuisine, used in tacos, salads, and as a topping.

12. Halloumi (Cyprus):

Taste and Texture: Halloumi is a semi-hard cheese with a unique, squeaky texture and a salty, briny flavor.

Uses: It’s great for grilling, frying, and serving in Mediterranean dishes.

These are just a few examples of the incredible diversity of cheese varieties available globally. Each cheese type brings its own distinct character to culinary creations, from appetizers to desserts, and reflects the rich cultural and regional traditions of its place of origin. Cheese enthusiasts can explore an extensive world of taste and texture by sampling various cheese varieties.

Artisanal vs. Industrial Cheese Production

The chapter will discuss the differences between artisanal and industrial cheese production. Readers will gain an appreciation for the skill and tradition in artisanal cheese-making and the efficiency and consistency in industrial production.

Cheese production can be broadly categorized into two main approaches: artisanal and industrial. Each method has its own unique characteristics, and the choice between them often depends on factors such as scale, tradition, and desired product consistency. Here's a comparison of artisanal and industrial cheese production:

Artisanal Cheese Production:

Scale: Artisanal cheese production is typically small-scale and often takes place on family farms or in small, independent creameries.

Hands-On: Artisanal cheese making is a labor-intensive, hands-on process that often relies on traditional, time-honored methods.

Ingredients: Artisanal producers often prioritize high-quality, local, and seasonal ingredients, including milk from a particular breed or from animals raised in specific conditions.

Variety: Artisanal producers may create a wide range of cheese varieties, often with unique flavors and characteristics based on local terroir.

Personalization: Artisanal producers have the flexibility to experiment with different recipes and adapt to changing consumer preferences, resulting in a level of personalization.

Production Time: The aging process for artisanal cheeses can be longer, resulting in complex flavors and textures.

Terroir: Artisanal cheese production often emphasizes the concept of terroir, where the local environment and climate influence the flavor and characteristics of the cheese.

Tradition: Artisanal cheese makers may adhere to traditional practices passed down through generations.

Industrial Cheese Production:

Scale: Industrial cheese production occurs on a much larger scale, often in large, mechanized facilities.

Automation: Industrial cheese production relies on automated machinery and standardized processes to increase efficiency and consistency.

Ingredients: Industrial cheese makers may use standardized, commercially available ingredients to achieve consistent results.

Consistency: Industrial cheese production aims for high consistency in flavor, texture, and appearance, making it possible to produce the same cheese variety with uniform characteristics across batches.

Standardization: Recipes and processes are standardized, allowing for mass production of popular cheese types.

Production Time: Industrial cheese production typically has shorter aging periods to meet consumer demand.

Efficiency: Industrial production is efficient and designed to meet the demands of a mass market.

Global Reach: Industrial cheese production enables the distribution of cheese varieties to a global market.

It's important to note that both artisanal and industrial cheese production have their place in the cheese industry. Artisanal cheese makers often focus on quality, diversity, and regional traditions, appealing to consumers who value unique and handmade products. Industrial cheese production, on the other hand, provides consistency, accessibility, and efficiency, making cheese varieties available to a broader consumer base.

Consumers' preferences vary, and they may appreciate both artisanal and industrial cheese for different occasions and culinary uses. Ultimately, the cheese-making approach chosen by a producer depends on their goals, available resources, and the market they aim to serve.

Cheese Maturation: The Aging Process

The aging of cheese is a critical aspect of its development. This section will explore the impact of time, temperature, and humidity on cheese maturation, resulting in the vast spectrum of flavors and textures in aged cheeses.

Cheese maturation, also known as cheese aging or affinage, is a critical phase in the production of many cheese varieties. During maturation, cheese undergoes complex biochemical and physical changes that lead to the development of its unique flavor, texture, and aroma. The aging process varies widely depending on the type of cheese being produced, but there are several common factors and stages in cheese maturation:

1. Curd Formation:

The maturation process begins during cheese production when the milk is coagulated, and curds are formed.

The texture, size, and moisture content of the curds at this stage will affect the cheese's final characteristics.

2. Brining or Salting:

Many cheeses are salted by immersing them in brine or by applying salt directly to the surface.

Salt enhances flavor, acts as a preservative, and helps to control the development of molds and bacteria.

3. Ripening Room:

After salting, the cheese is moved to ripening rooms with controlled temperature and humidity.

The conditions in these rooms play a significant role in shaping the cheese's characteristics.

4. Microbial Activity:

The cheese undergoes complex biochemical changes due to the activity of various microorganisms, such as bacteria and molds.

These microorganisms contribute to flavor development, texture changes, and the formation of rind or natural coatings.

5. Protein and Fat Breakdown:

During maturation, enzymes break down proteins and fats, which contributes to flavor and texture changes.

Proteolysis (protein breakdown) and lipolysis (fat breakdown) can lead to the creation of amino acids, fatty acids, and other compounds that influence the cheese's taste.

6. Aroma Development:

As cheese matures, various compounds are produced or released, contributing to its aroma.

These compounds can include esters, aldehydes, and sulfur compounds that give the cheese its characteristic scent.

7. Texture Changes:

The texture of the cheese evolves during maturation due to moisture loss and the breakdown of proteins and fats.

Aging can lead to a firmer, crumbly texture in some cheeses and a creamier, smoother texture in others.

8. Rind Formation:

Some cheeses develop a natural rind, which can be influenced by molds or bacteria present in the ripening environment.

The rind can contribute to the cheese's flavor and appearance.

9. Aging Duration:

The duration of maturation varies greatly, from just a few weeks for some fresh cheeses to several years for aged and extra-aged varieties.

The cheese maker carefully monitors the aging process and determines when the cheese has reached its peak quality.

10. Quality Assessment:

Experienced cheese makers may assess the cheese's quality during maturation by using sensory evaluation or analytical methods to ensure it meets the desired characteristics.

The maturation process is a delicate balance of time, temperature, humidity, and microbial activity. Each cheese variety requires its specific maturation conditions to achieve its unique taste and texture. Whether it's the crumbly texture of aged Parmesan, the creamy interior of a Brie, or the blue veins of Roquefort, cheese maturation is the art and science behind creating a world of diverse and delightful cheese varieties.

Cheese and Terroir

The concept of terroir, which is deeply rooted in the world of wine, plays a significant role in cheese production. Readers will understand how the environment, from the soil to the climate, influences the characteristics of cheese, giving rise to unique regional flavors.

Terroir is a concept typically associated with wine and is used to describe how the environment and local factors influence the flavor and characteristics of agricultural products. While terroir is most commonly applied to grapes and the production of wine, it can also play a role in the production of cheese. Here's how terroir impacts cheese production:

Milk Source: The primary ingredient in cheese is milk, and the source of this milk can have a significant impact on the final product. The diet and forage available to dairy animals, as well as the local climate, all contribute to the unique flavor profile of the milk. For example, cows grazing on Alpine pastures produce milk that is ideal for the production of Alpine-style cheeses like Gruyère.

Local Flora: The environment in which the animals graze affects the microbial and bacterial flora present in the milk. Local microflora play a critical role in cheese production by contributing to fermentation and influencing the flavor and texture of the cheese. For example, the microflora found in the air and on the vegetation in the region can be crucial in the production of specific cheese varieties.

Altitude and Climate: The altitude at which the animals are raised and the local climate have an impact on the quality and composition of the milk. For instance, in Alpine regions, the cooler temperatures and fresh mountain air can lead to a different milk composition, which results in distinct flavors in the cheese.

Geography and Soil Composition: The geography and soil composition of the region can influence the types of vegetation and forage available to dairy animals. The minerals and nutrients absorbed by the plants can, in turn, be present in the milk and affect the cheese's flavor and texture.

Traditional Production Methods: Local cheese-making traditions and techniques, passed down through generations, are also part of the terroir. These methods reflect the history and culture of the region and are integral to the production of specific cheese varieties.

Terroir plays a significant role in the production of various artisanal and traditional cheeses. It is particularly evident in the production of regional and specialty cheeses, such as Roquefort from France, Parmigiano-Reggiano from Italy, or Stilton from England. The concept of terroir helps consumers understand and appreciate the unique qualities of these cheeses, which are deeply rooted in their places of origin.

Overall, terroir is a critical aspect of artisanal cheese production, emphasizing the connection between the environment, tradition, and the end product's distinct flavor and characteristics.

The Culinary Versatility of Cheese

Cheese is a culinary chameleon, and this section will explore its versatility in various cuisines. Readers will discover how cheese can elevate dishes, from the Italian tradition of pairing mozzarella with tomatoes to the French love affair with creamy Brie.

Cheese is renowned for its incredible culinary versatility. It can be a star ingredient in a wide range of dishes or serve as a complementary component to enhance flavor, texture, and visual appeal. Here are some of the many ways cheese can be used in the culinary world:

Cheese Boards and Platters: Cheese boards are a popular appetizer or snack option. They typically feature an array of cheeses, along with accompaniments like crackers, fruits, nuts, and charcuterie. A well-arranged cheese board can be a visually stunning and delicious addition to any gathering.

Grating and Melting: Grated cheese is a versatile topping for pasta, pizzas, casseroles, and salads. Melting cheese, such as mozzarella, cheddar, or

Swiss, adds a creamy and savory element to dishes like lasagna, grilled cheese sandwiches, and fondue.

Sandwiches and Wraps: Cheese can elevate a sandwich to a whole new level. Whether it's the classic grilled cheese, a gourmet panini, or a veggie wrap, cheese adds a rich and flavorful component to many sandwich creations.

Salads: Cheese, especially varieties like feta, goat cheese, or blue cheese, can provide a tangy and creamy contrast to the freshness of salads. Cheese crumbles or shavings can be used to enhance both the taste and presentation of salads.

Appetizers and Hors d'Oeuvres: Cheese is a staple of appetizer menus. It can be incorporated into items like stuffed mushrooms, cheese-stuffed jalapeños, or bite-sized cheese balls or croquettes.

Dips and Sauces: Cheese is a key ingredient in many dips and sauces. Queso dip, spinach and artichoke dip, and a classic cheese sauce for macaroni and cheese are just a few examples.

Desserts: While cheese is often associated with savory dishes, it also plays a role in sweet treats. Cream cheese is a fundamental component of cheesecakes, and ricotta cheese is used in cannoli filling. There are even dessert cheeses, like mascarpone, that are used in various confections.

Pairing with Wine and Fruit: Cheese pairs exceptionally well with wine, and the right combination can create a delightful sensory experience. Popular pairings include red wine with cheddar or Port wine with blue cheese. Cheese also complements a variety of fruits, such as apples, pears, and grapes.

Omelettes and Quiches: Cheese adds depth and creaminess to omelettes and quiches. Varieties like Swiss, feta, or goat cheese can be mixed with eggs and a range of ingredients for a satisfying breakfast or brunch option.

International Cuisine: Cheese is used in diverse international cuisines. Think of paneer in Indian dishes, halloumi in Mediterranean cuisine, or queso fresco in Latin American fare. Each cheese brings its unique character to these culinary traditions.

Baking and Pastry: Cheese can be incorporated into baking, adding a savory twist to items like cheese scones, cheese straws, and savory tarts.

Toppings and Condiments: Cheese can be grated or crumbled as a topping for soups, chili, or baked potatoes. It's also a common addition to burgers and hot dogs, where it adds flavor and richness.

The culinary versatility of cheese knows no bounds, making it a beloved ingredient in kitchens around the world. Whether you're creating comfort food, gourmet cuisine, or exploring new flavor combinations, cheese is a versatile and delicious addition to your culinary repertoire.

Cheese in Appetizers and Main Courses

The section will delve into the role of cheese in appetizers and main courses. Readers will learn how cheese can be featured in a variety of culinary creations, from stuffed mushrooms to lasagna and quiches.

Cheese is a versatile ingredient that can be used in a wide range of appetizers and main courses. Its rich and savory flavors can enhance various dishes, adding depth and creaminess. Here are some appetizer and main course ideas that feature cheese:

Appetizers:

Stuffed Mushrooms: Create a filling with cream cheese, garlic, herbs, and grated Parmesan, then stuff mushroom caps. Bake until the mushrooms are tender and the filling is golden brown.

Cheese Fondue: Prepare a classic cheese fondue by melting a mixture of Swiss and Gruyère cheese with white wine and a touch of kirsch. Serve with bread cubes, vegetables, and cured meats for dipping.

Caprese Skewers: Skewer cherry tomatoes, fresh basil leaves, and bite-sized mozzarella balls. Drizzle with balsamic glaze and olive oil, then season with salt and pepper.

Spinach and Artichoke Dip: Make a creamy dip with cream cheese, sour cream, grated Parmesan, and chopped spinach and artichoke hearts. Serve with tortilla chips, pita bread, or vegetable sticks.

Baked Brie: Encase a wheel of Brie in puff pastry, add fruit preserves or honey, and bake until the pastry is golden and the cheese is gooey. Serve with crackers or sliced baguette.

Mini Quiches: Create bite-sized quiches with a savory pastry crust filled with a mixture of eggs, cream, cheese, and various ingredients like bacon, spinach, or mushrooms.

Cheese Straws: Make flaky pastry straws by folding grated cheese into puff pastry, then cutting and twisting the dough. Bake until golden and crispy.

Main Courses:

Macaroni and Cheese: Prepare a creamy cheese sauce with a blend of cheddar, mozzarella, and Parmesan. Toss it with cooked macaroni for a classic comfort food dish.

Lasagna: Layer lasagna noodles with ricotta, mozzarella, Parmesan, and a rich tomato sauce. Bake until bubbly and golden.

Chicken Alfredo: Create a velvety Alfredo sauce with butter, cream, and grated Parmesan. Serve over grilled or sautéed chicken breast and fettuccine pasta.

Cheese-Stuffed Burgers: Make juicy burgers with a surprise in the center—cheese! Form ground beef or turkey patties around cubes of cheddar, Swiss, or blue cheese.

Vegetable Gratin: Layer sliced vegetables like potatoes or zucchini with a creamy cheese sauce. Bake until the vegetables are tender and the top is golden brown.

Pizza: Top pizza dough with tomato sauce, mozzarella cheese, and various toppings of your choice, such as pepperoni, vegetables, or sausage.

Spinach and Feta Stuffed Chicken: Cut a pocket in boneless, skinless chicken breasts and stuff them with a mixture of spinach, feta cheese, and herbs. Bake until the chicken is cooked through.

Grilled Cheese Sandwiches: Create gourmet grilled cheese sandwiches by adding different cheeses and ingredients like bacon, caramelized onions, or sliced tomatoes.

Cheese and Vegetable Quesadillas: Layer tortillas with a mixture of grated cheese, sautéed vegetables, and your choice of protein. Cook until the tortillas are crispy and the cheese is melted.

These are just a few examples of how cheese can be incorporated into appetizers and main courses. With the wide variety of cheeses available, you can experiment with different flavors and textures to create dishes that suit your taste and culinary preferences.

The Cultural Significance of Cheese

The chapter will highlight the cultural significance of cheese in various regions. Readers will appreciate the deep traditions, celebrations, and rituals associated with cheese in countries like France, Italy, and Switzerland.

Cheese holds immense cultural significance in various societies around the world. Its role goes beyond mere sustenance; it is deeply embedded in traditions, customs, and culinary heritage. Here's a glimpse of the cultural significance of cheese:

1. France - The Land of 1,000 Cheeses: France is renowned for its cheese culture, boasting over 1,000 distinct varieties of cheese. French cheeses like Brie, Camembert, and Roquefort are celebrated for their regional origins, and the French take great pride in their cheese-making traditions. Cheese and wine pairings are a cherished aspect of French cuisine.

2. Italy - The Home of Mozzarella and Parmesan: Italy is famous for its iconic cheeses, including Mozzarella, Parmigiano-Reggiano, and Pecorino Romano. These cheeses are integral to Italian culinary culture and are essential ingredients in dishes like pizza, pasta, and risotto.

3. Greece - Feta and Beyond: Feta cheese is a cornerstone of Greek cuisine, used in Greek salads, pastries, and as a garnish for many dishes. The role of cheese in Greek culture extends to religious traditions, such as the custom of breaking cheese during Easter.

4. Switzerland - Swiss Cheese and Fondue: Swiss cheese varieties, like Emmental and Gruyère, are internationally renowned. The fondue, a communal melted cheese dish, is an integral part of Swiss culture, bringing people together for warm and convivial gatherings.

5. Mexico - Queso Fresco and Cotija: Mexican cuisine features various cheeses, including Queso Fresco and Cotija. These cheeses are used in dishes like tacos, enchiladas, and tamales, contributing to the unique flavors of Mexican food.

6. The United Kingdom - Cheddar and Stilton: Cheese plays a significant role in British cuisine. Cheddar and Stilton are iconic British cheeses, and cheese ploughman's lunches are a classic pub dish. Cheese rolling competitions, like the Cooper's Hill Cheese-Rolling and Wake, are popular cultural events.

7. India - Paneer and Chhena: Paneer, a fresh cheese, is a staple in Indian vegetarian cuisine. It is used in a variety of curries, desserts, and snacks. Chhena, another form of fresh cheese, is used in Indian sweets like rasgulla and sandesh.

8. The Netherlands - Gouda and Edam: The Netherlands is renowned for its cheese production,

with Gouda and Edam being well-known Dutch cheese varieties. Cheese markets in cities like Alkmaar are cultural attractions, offering a glimpse into the country's cheese heritage.

9. Switzerland - Swiss Cheese and Fondue: Swiss cheese varieties, like Emmental and Gruyère, are internationally renowned. The fondue, a communal melted cheese dish, is an integral part of Swiss culture, bringing people together for warm and convivial gatherings.

10. Greece - Feta and Beyond: Feta cheese is a cornerstone of Greek cuisine, used in Greek salads, pastries, and as a garnish for many dishes. The role of cheese in Greek culture extends to religious traditions, such as the custom of breaking cheese during Easter.

11. Japan - Cheese in Modern Cuisine: While cheese is not a traditional Japanese food, it has found its place in modern Japanese cuisine. Items like cheese-filled pastries and cheese-topped dishes have gained popularity.

12. The United States - American Cheese and Beyond: The United States has a diverse cheese culture, with a growing number of artisanal cheese

producers. American cheese, known for its melting qualities, is widely used in burgers and sandwiches.

Cheese is not just a source of nourishment but also a symbol of heritage and identity. It is a bridge between generations, an emblem of regional pride, and a delightful avenue for cultural exchange. As people share their cheese traditions, they also share their stories, values, and history. The cultural significance of cheese is a testament to its enduring role in our collective culinary experience.

Innovation and Trends in Cheese

The chapter will conclude with a look at innovation and trends in the cheese industry. Readers will gain insight into modern cheese-making techniques, the rise of artisanal cheese, and the evolving preferences of cheese connoisseurs.

The cheese industry is continually evolving with innovations and emerging trends. These developments are driven by consumer preferences, technological advancements, sustainability concerns, and a desire to create new and exciting cheese products. Here are some of the innovation and trends in the world of cheese:

1. Artisanal and Craft Cheeses: Consumers are increasingly interested in unique, handcrafted

cheeses made by local artisans. These cheeses often showcase traditional production methods and regional flavors, emphasizing quality over quantity.

2. Plant-Based and Vegan Cheeses: The demand for plant-based and vegan alternatives to dairy products has grown significantly. Innovations in plant-based cheese production have resulted in products that closely mimic the taste and texture of traditional cheese.

3. Ethnic and Global Flavors: Cheese producers are exploring a wide range of global flavors and ingredients to create fusion cheeses. This trend allows consumers to explore different cultural tastes within the context of cheese.

4. Sustainable Cheese Production: Sustainability is a growing concern in the cheese industry. Some producers are adopting eco-friendly practices, such as using renewable energy, reducing waste, and minimizing water usage.

5. Cheese Aging and Affinage: The practice of cheese aging and affinage is becoming more sophisticated. Affineurs (cheese agers) are experimenting with different aging conditions, such as temperature and humidity, to develop unique cheese profiles.

6. Health-Conscious Cheese Products: Cheese with added health benefits, such as probiotics or lower salt content, is gaining traction. These products cater to health-conscious consumers looking for nutritious cheese options.

7. Novel Cheese Blends: Cheese makers are creating innovative blends of different cheese varieties, combining flavors, textures, and colors to offer unique cheese experiences.

8. Cheese and Beverage Pairings: The art of pairing cheese with various beverages, including wine, craft beer, and cider, is becoming more popular. This trend encourages consumers to explore complementary flavor profiles.

9. Cheese Snacking: Cheese snacks, such as cheese sticks, cheese crisps, and portable cheese portions, have gained popularity as convenient and protein-rich on-the-go options.

10. Reduced Packaging Waste: Cheese producers are adopting more sustainable packaging options, such as recyclable and biodegradable materials, as well as portion control packaging to reduce food waste.

11. Cheese Subscription Services: Cheese subscription services allow consumers to discover

new and unique cheeses regularly, delivered directly to their door.

12. Cheese Tourism: Cheese-related tourism, including visits to cheese dairies, creameries, and cheese festivals, has become a popular way for enthusiasts to learn about cheese production and taste local varieties.

13. Digital Cheese Education: The use of online platforms, including websites and social media, to educate consumers about cheese, its history, and how to pair it with various foods and beverages has become more prevalent.

14. Redefining Cheese Norms: Innovators are redefining what cheese can be. Examples include "bread cheese" that can be grilled, "smoked" cheese made with smoked water, and "crystal cheese" with a crunchy texture.

15. Traditional Revival: In some regions, there's a revival of traditional and historical cheese recipes, breathing new life into heritage varieties.

The cheese industry continues to adapt and evolve to meet changing consumer preferences and environmental concerns. These trends and innovations are shaping the future of cheese, making it an exciting and dynamic field within the food industry.

The Role of Microbes in Cheese

Microbes, such as bacteria and molds, play a pivotal role in cheese development. This section will provide a deeper understanding of how specific microbial strains are harnessed to create the wide range of flavors and textures found in cheese.

Microbes play a fundamental role in cheese production, contributing to the flavor, texture, and safety of the final product. Here's an overview of the key ways in which microbes are involved in the cheese-making process:

Starter Cultures: Starter cultures are a mix of specific lactic acid bacteria (LAB) used to acidify milk during cheese production. These bacteria convert lactose (milk sugar) into lactic acid, which lowers the pH of the milk. This acidification is crucial for coagulating the milk and forming curds. Common LAB used in starter cultures include Lactococcus, Streptococcus, and Lactobacillus species.

Acidification: The starter cultures play a critical role in the acidification of milk, which is necessary for the coagulation of proteins and the development of cheese curds. The rate and extent of acid production by LAB contribute to the cheese's texture and flavor.

Ripening and Flavor Development: During cheese ripening or aging, various bacteria, molds, and yeasts are introduced to the cheese. These microbes metabolize residual lactose and other nutrients, producing a wide range of flavor compounds. For example, propionic acid bacteria are responsible for the characteristic nutty flavor of Swiss cheese, while Penicillium molds contribute to the blue veins in blue cheese.

Texture and Aroma: Microbes can influence the texture of cheese. Some bacteria, such as Brevibacterium linens, contribute to the development of a natural rind on certain cheeses and can influence aroma and flavor. These surface-ripened cheeses are often soft and pungent.

Protection from Spoilage: Beneficial bacteria and molds can protect cheese from spoilage microorganisms. By occupying space and consuming nutrients, these desirable microbes prevent the growth of harmful bacteria and molds.

Safety and Shelf-Life: The controlled use of specific bacterial cultures contributes to the safety and shelf-life of cheese. LAB produce lactic acid, which lowers the pH of the cheese, creating an environment that inhibits the growth of harmful pathogens.

Proteolysis: Microbes are also involved in the breakdown of proteins in cheese. This process, known as proteolysis, is responsible for the development of complex flavors and aromas in aged cheeses.

Texture and Mouthfeel: Microbes can influence the texture and mouthfeel of cheese. In some varieties, they produce enzymes that break down proteins, leading to a smoother and creamier texture.

Surface-ripened Cheeses: For cheeses like Brie and Camembert, specific molds and yeasts are essential. These surface-ripened cheeses develop their characteristic white, fluffy rinds and soft, creamy interiors through the actions of these microbes.

Washed-rind Cheeses: Cheeses like Limburger and Munster are known for their pungent aroma and distinctive orange or pink rinds, which are developed through the action of specific bacteria.

These bacteria contribute to the cheese's unique character.

Blue-veined Cheeses: In blue cheese varieties like Roquefort and Gorgonzola, molds (Penicillium roqueforti or Penicillium glaucum) are intentionally introduced. The blue veins result from the growth of these molds throughout the cheese.

Microbes are an integral part of cheese production and are carefully selected and managed by cheese makers to achieve the desired characteristics and quality in each cheese variety. The diversity of microbes used in cheese production contributes to the immense variety of flavors, textures, and appearances found in the world of cheese.

The Culinary Diversity of Cheese

The chapter will continue by delving into the culinary diversity of cheese, highlighting its roles in appetizers, salads, main courses, and desserts. Readers will gain a deeper appreciation for the myriad ways in which cheese can be incorporated into dishes.

Cheese is a remarkably versatile ingredient in the culinary world, and its diverse range of flavors, textures, and melting properties makes it a favorite in many cuisines. Here are some examples of the culinary diversity of cheese:

1. Italian Cuisine:

Parmesan: Grated Parmesan is a staple for pasta dishes like spaghetti and lasagna.

Mozzarella: Fresh mozzarella is used in Caprese salads, while shredded mozzarella is a must for pizzas.

Gorgonzola: Gorgonzola cheese adds depth and creaminess to risottos and salads.

2. French Cuisine:

Brie: Brie is often enjoyed with fresh baguettes and fruit, and it can be baked en croûte for a decadent appetizer.

Camembert: Like Brie, Camembert is excellent for spreading on crackers or crusty bread.

Roquefort: Roquefort cheese is a key ingredient in classic French dishes like quiches and salads.

3. Swiss Cuisine:

Emmental and Gruyère: These Swiss cheeses are essential for traditional dishes like fondue and raclette.

4. Mexican Cuisine:

Queso Fresco: Queso fresco is often crumbled over tacos, salads, and beans.

Queso Blanco: Queso blanco is used in Mexican dishes like chiles rellenos and enchiladas.

5. American Cuisine:

Cheddar: Cheddar cheese is widely used in burgers, grilled cheese sandwiches, and macaroni and cheese.

Cream Cheese: Cream cheese is the base for cheesecakes, and it's often spread on bagels.

6. Mediterranean Cuisine:

Feta: Feta cheese is a key ingredient in Greek salads and spanakopita.

Halloumi: Halloumi cheese is often grilled and served in Mediterranean salads or as a side dish.

7. Indian Cuisine:

Paneer: Paneer is used in a variety of Indian dishes, including saag paneer and paneer tikka.

8. Middle Eastern Cuisine:

Labneh: Labneh, a strained yogurt cheese, is used as a spread or dip.

Akawi: Akawi cheese is common in Middle Eastern pastries and desserts.

9. Japanese Cuisine:

Cream Cheese (in Sushi): Cream cheese is used in some sushi rolls, like the Philadelphia roll.

Yakiguni: Yakiguni cheese is sometimes added to Japanese curry dishes.

10. Eastern European Cuisine:

Pierogi Fillings: In Eastern European cuisine, cheese fillings for pierogi are popular, such as potato and cheese or sweet cheese pierogi.

11. Southern Cuisine:

Pimento Cheese: Pimento cheese is a Southern staple often served as a spread or dip, as well as in sandwiches.

12. Swiss Cuisine:

Appenzeller: Appenzeller cheese is used in Swiss-style rosti (potato fritters) and fondue.

13. Korean Cuisine:

Tteokbokki with Cheese: In Korean cuisine, tteokbokki (spicy rice cakes) with added cheese has become a popular street food.

These are just a few examples of the culinary diversity of cheese. Cheese's adaptability and ability to enhance a wide range of dishes make it a beloved ingredient worldwide. From savory to sweet, cheese is an essential component of many cuisines, adding rich flavors, creamy textures, and depth to a multitude of dishes.

Pairing Cheese with Wine and Beyond

Pairing cheese with beverages is an art in itself. This section will provide guidance on pairing cheese with wines, beers, and other accompaniments, enhancing the overall tasting experience.

Pairing cheese with wine, beer, and other beverages is a delightful culinary experience that enhances the flavors of both the cheese and the drink. Here are some tips and ideas for pairing cheese with various beverages:

1. Wine and Cheese Pairing:

Red Wine: Robust, aged cheeses like Cheddar, Gouda, and Parmesan pair well with red wines like Cabernet Sauvignon and Merlot.

White Wine: Light and fresh cheeses like Brie, Camembert, and goat cheese complement white wines such as Chardonnay and Sauvignon Blanc.

Rosé Wine: Mild, semi-soft cheeses like Gruyère and Emmental are a good match for rosé wines.

Sparkling Wine: Creamy, soft cheeses like Triple Crème Brie and Camembert go wonderfully with sparkling wines like Champagne.

Port Wine: Stilton and Roquefort cheeses pair perfectly with the sweetness of Port wine.

2. Beer and Cheese Pairing:

Pilsner or Lager: Light and crisp beers like pilsner or lager are excellent with milder cheeses like mozzarella, Colby, and Monterey Jack.

IPA (India Pale Ale): The hoppy bitterness of an IPA pairs well with strong, sharp cheeses like cheddar and blue cheese.

Stout: Rich and creamy stouts complement robust cheeses such as Gouda and Parmesan.

Wheat Beer: Wheat beer pairs nicely with soft and creamy cheeses, including brie and Camembert.

3. Whiskey and Cheese Pairing:

Bourbon: The sweetness and caramel notes of bourbon complement semi-hard cheeses like Cheddar and Comté.

Scotch: The smoky and peaty flavors of Scotch whisky can pair well with strong, pungent cheeses like blue cheese and gorgonzola.

Irish Whiskey: The smoothness of Irish whiskey is an excellent match for milder cheeses like havarti and fontina.

4. Coffee and Cheese Pairing:

Espresso: The bold and robust flavor of espresso pairs with hard, aged cheeses like Parmigiano-Reggiano and Pecorino Romano.

Cappuccino: The creamy texture of cappuccino goes well with creamy cheeses like gouda and camembert.

Cold Brew: Cold brew coffee's smooth and slightly sweet profile complements soft, mild cheeses like mozzarella and brie.

5. Tea and Cheese Pairing:

Black Tea: Black teas with bold flavors, such as Darjeeling or Assam, pair nicely with strong cheeses like cheddar and gorgonzola.

Green Tea: Light and grassy green teas work well with delicate cheeses like goat cheese and feta.

Herbal Tea: Herbal teas like chamomile or peppermint can be paired with fresh and mild cheeses like mozzarella and ricotta.

6. Fruit Juice and Cheese Pairing:

Apple Juice: The crispness of apple juice complements cheddar and other hard cheeses.

Pear Juice: The sweetness and subtle pear flavor pair nicely with blue cheese and Camembert.

Grape Juice: The natural sweetness of grape juice is great with mild cheeses like havarti and gouda.

When pairing cheese with beverages, consider the intensity and flavor profile of both the cheese and the drink. Experiment with different combinations to discover your personal preferences. The key is to enjoy the delightful interplay of flavors and textures that arise from these pairings.

CHAPTER SEVEN

Butter, Cream, and All Things Rich

Butter and cream, known for their luxurious richness and delectable flavors, have a special place in the world of dairy. In this chapter, we'll explore the art of butter and cream production, their culinary significance, and their role in enhancing the flavors of various dishes.

The Allure of Butter

The chapter will begin by discussing the timeless allure of butter. Readers will gain an appreciation for the creamy, rich taste of butter, its versatility in cooking, and its cultural significance in culinary traditions.

Butter is a beloved and versatile ingredient in cooking and baking. Its rich, creamy, and savory qualities make it a staple in many cuisines and recipes. Here's a closer look at the allure of butter:

1. Flavor Enhancement:

Richness: Butter adds a luxurious, rich flavor to dishes. It enhances the taste of everything it's added to, from vegetables and grains to meats and seafood.

Nutty and Slightly Sweet: When butter is browned, it takes on a nutty and slightly sweet flavor that adds depth to both savory and sweet dishes.

Aromatics: Butter is often used as a base for sautéing or sweating aromatics like onions and garlic, infusing them with a delightful flavor.

2. Versatility:

Cooking: Butter is used for sautéing, frying, and pan-searing. It's essential for making sauces and gravies, such as béchamel and hollandaise.

Baking: Butter is a primary ingredient in many baked goods, including cookies, cakes, pastries, and pie crusts. It contributes to the tender and flaky texture of pastries.

Finishing: A pat of butter can be added to a hot dish just before serving to enrich its taste and create a glossy finish.

Compound Butter: Butter can be infused with various ingredients like herbs, spices, and citrus zest to create compound butter for flavoring dishes or as a condiment.

3. Texture and Mouthfeel:

Creaminess: Butter adds a creamy and silky texture to dishes. This is especially important in sauces, mashed potatoes, and risottos.

Emulsification: In emulsified sauces like hollandaise, the fat in butter plays a crucial role in creating a smooth and stable texture.

4. Baking Essential:

Pastry Dough: Butter is a key ingredient in making flaky and tender pie crusts, puff pastry, and croissants.

Leavening: In baking, butter can be creamed with sugar to trap air, contributing to the leavening of cakes and cookies.

5. Shelf Life:

Longevity: Butter has a relatively long shelf life when refrigerated, making it a handy ingredient for home cooks.

Freezing: It can also be frozen for even longer storage.

6. Cultural Significance:

Cultural Traditions: Butter holds cultural significance in various cuisines. For example, ghee (clarified butter) is a staple in Indian cooking, while French cuisine relies on butter for its rich sauces.

Holiday and Festive Dishes: Many holiday and festive dishes, such as Christmas cookies and Thanksgiving stuffing, call for generous amounts of butter.

7. Natural and Simple Ingredient:

Minimal Processing: Butter is typically made from cream that is churned to separate the fat from the liquid. It's a natural and minimally processed product.

Transcends Generations: Butter has been a staple in cooking for generations, connecting past traditions with modern recipes.

8. Flavor Pairings:

Salted Butter: Salted butter complements both sweet and savory dishes. It's often spread on bread or used to finish vegetables and meats.

Unsalted Butter: Unsalted butter allows for more precise control of salt in recipes, making it ideal for baking and many cooking applications.

9. Ingredient in Classic Dishes:

Beurre Blanc: A classic French sauce made with butter, white wine, and shallots.

Beurre Noisette: Browned butter used in both savory and sweet dishes.

Butter's allure lies in its ability to transform and elevate the flavors and textures of a wide range of dishes, making it a cherished ingredient for both professional chefs and home cooks. Whether used to sauté vegetables, enrich sauces, or create flaky pastries, butter is a culinary essential with timeless appeal.

Butter Making: From Cream to Gold

The process of butter making will be explored in detail. Readers will understand how cream is churned to separate the butterfat from the buttermilk, resulting in the creation of golden, flavorful butter.

The process of making butter from cream is a simple yet fascinating journey from a liquid dairy product to a spreadable or semi-solid delight. Here is an overview of how butter is made:

1. Sourcing Cream:

Cream is the primary ingredient in butter production. It can be sourced from cow's milk and can vary in fat content, with heavy cream or double cream being ideal for butter making.

2. Separation:

In traditional butter making, cream is allowed to sit undisturbed, which causes the fat molecules to separate from the liquid. This process is known as cream separation.

3. Churning:

The separated cream is then churned, either through traditional methods like a butter churn or mechanically using a butter churner. The churning process agitates the cream, causing the fat molecules to clump together.

4. Formation of Butter Grains:

As churning continues, the fat molecules cluster together and form solid particles. These solid particles are the butter grains or butter curd.

5. Separation of Butter and Buttermilk:

The continuous churning causes the butter grains to separate from the remaining liquid, which is now buttermilk. The buttermilk can be drained off, leaving behind the butter grains.

6. Washing and Kneading:

The butter grains are often washed with cold water to remove any remaining buttermilk, which can spoil the butter. After washing, the butter is kneaded to remove excess moisture.

7. Salt (Optional):

If desired, salt can be added to the butter during the kneading process. Salt enhances the flavor and acts as a preservative.

8. Shaping and Packaging:

The butter is shaped into blocks, pats, or rolls. It can be wrapped in parchment paper or placed in containers for packaging.

9. Storage:

The freshly made butter should be stored in a cool, dry place or in the refrigerator to maintain its freshness.

It's important to note that while traditional butter making involves churning, modern butter production often utilizes cream separators and centrifuges to separate the fat from the liquid. However, the basic principle of fat separation remains the same.

Butter can be enjoyed as a spread on bread, used in cooking and baking, or as a flavorful addition to various dishes. Its creamy texture and rich, savory flavor make it a staple in many kitchens worldwide.

Types of Butter

The chapter will delve into the various types of butter, from the classic unsalted and salted varieties to specialty butters infused with herbs, spices, and other flavorings. Readers will learn how different types of butter can elevate dishes.

Butter comes in various types, each with distinct characteristics, flavors, and uses. Here are some of the most common types of butter:

1. Unsalted Butter:

Unsalted butter, as the name suggests, does not contain added salt. It's a versatile butter used in both cooking and baking. Since it doesn't have added salt, it allows for more precise control of salt levels in recipes.

2. Salted Butter:

Salted butter contains added salt, typically in small amounts. It's often used as a spread on bread or toast and can also be used in cooking and baking. The salt enhances the flavor and acts as a natural preservative.

3. Clarified Butter (Ghee):

Clarified butter, often referred to as ghee in Indian cuisine, is made by melting regular butter and separating the liquid fat from the milk solids and water. Ghee has a high smoke point and a rich, nutty flavor. It is commonly used in Indian cooking and is also suitable for frying and sautéing.

4. European-Style Butter:

European-style butter is known for its higher fat content and lower water content compared to regular butter. It has a creamier texture and a richer flavor, making it ideal for baking, pastry making, and for spreading on bread.

5. Cultured Butter:

Cultured butter is made from cream that has been fermented with beneficial bacteria before churning. This process gives the butter a tangy flavor and a creamy texture. It's excellent for spreading on bread or enhancing the flavor of dishes.

6. Grass-Fed Butter:

Butter made from the milk of grass-fed cows is known for its rich and distinctive flavor. The diet of the cows contributes to the butter's unique taste. It's often sought after by those looking for a more natural and flavorful option.

7. Flavored Butter:

Flavored butter is created by mixing butter with various ingredients such as herbs, spices, garlic, or citrus zest. It's used to add flavor to dishes, especially when finishing or garnishing. Common examples include garlic butter, herb butter, and lemon butter.

8. Whipped Butter:

Whipped butter is regular butter that has been whipped to incorporate air, making it easier to spread. It has a lighter texture and is suitable for spreading on bread and rolls.

9. Vegan Butter:

Vegan butter is a plant-based alternative to dairy butter. It's made from vegetable oils, such as soybean or coconut oil, and often includes emulsifiers and flavorings to mimic the taste and texture of dairy butter. Vegan butter is suitable for individuals who follow a vegan or lactose-free diet.

10. Specialty Butter:

Specialty butters include unique varieties like truffle butter, brown butter (beurre noisette), and compound butters, which are butter blends infused with herbs, spices, or other flavorings. These specialty butters are used to add distinct and luxurious flavors to dishes.

The choice of butter type depends on your culinary needs and personal preferences. Whether you're sautéing, baking, or spreading it on your morning toast, there's a type of butter that's perfectly suited to the task.

Cooking with Butter

Readers will explore the culinary uses of butter, from sautéing and frying to baking. This section will provide insights into how butter enhances flavors, textures, and aromas in a wide range of dishes.

Cooking with butter can add a rich and savory flavor to your dishes. Here are some tips and techniques for cooking with butter:

1. Sautéing and Frying:

Butter is excellent for sautéing vegetables and aromatics. It adds a depth of flavor to dishes like sautéed mushrooms or onions.

It can be used for pan-frying chicken, fish, or pork chops, providing a deliciously crispy exterior.

2. Making Sauces:

Butter is a key ingredient in many classic sauces, such as béchamel, hollandaise, and lemon butter sauce.

To make a simple pan sauce, deglaze the pan with wine, broth, or other liquids, and then swirl in a knob of butter to add richness and create a silky texture.

3. Baking:

Butter is a staple in baking and is used to make cookies, cakes, pastries, and pie crusts. It provides flavor, moisture, and a tender texture to baked goods.

4. Flavoring and Finishing:

A pat of butter can be added to hot dishes just before serving to enhance flavor and create a glossy finish. This is known as "mounting" the dish with butter.

Compound butter, which is butter blended with herbs, spices, or other flavorings, can be used to add a burst of flavor to dishes. It's especially great for grilled meats, vegetables, or hot bread.

5. Brown Butter (Beurre Noisette):

To make brown butter, melt butter in a pan over medium heat and let it cook until it turns golden brown and develops a nutty aroma. It's a delicious addition to dishes like pasta, gnocchi, and vegetables.

6. Clarified Butter (Ghee):

Clarified butter has a high smoke point and is ideal for high-heat cooking methods like frying or searing. It's commonly used in Indian cuisine.

7. Cooking Tips:

When sautéing, be mindful of not letting the butter brown too much or burn, as it can develop a bitter taste. You can add a small amount of oil to the pan to help prevent this.

Use unsalted butter when you want to control the salt content in your dishes. Add salt to taste, as needed.

8. Substituting Butter:

In some recipes, you can substitute other fats like olive oil, coconut oil, or vegetable oil for butter. However, be aware that these substitutions can change the flavor and texture of the dish.

9. Brown Butter for Sweet and Savory Dishes:

Brown butter can be used in both sweet and savory recipes. It adds a nutty, caramelized flavor to dishes like roasted vegetables, pasta, or brown butter cookies.

Cooking with butter adds a wonderful richness and depth of flavor to a wide range of dishes. Experiment with different cooking methods and butter types to discover the perfect combination for your favorite recipes.

Cultured Butter: A Delicacy

Cultured butter, often favored for its tangy depth of flavor, will be examined. Readers will understand the role of bacterial cultures in the fermentation process and how it contributes to the distinct taste of cultured butter.

Cultured butter, often considered a delicacy, is a type of butter made from cream that has been fermented with beneficial bacteria before churning. This process gives cultured butter its unique and desirable characteristics. Here's what you need to know about this flavorful butter:

1. Tangy Flavor:

Cultured butter has a distinct tangy and slightly nutty flavor. This tanginess comes from the fermentation of the cream by lactic acid bacteria, which convert lactose into lactic acid.

2. Creamy Texture:

Cultured butter is known for its creamy and smooth texture. It spreads easily and melts beautifully, making it a perfect choice for topping warm bread or muffins.

3. Versatile:

It's a versatile butter suitable for a wide range of culinary applications. You can use it for cooking, baking, or as a condiment.

4. High Fat Content:

Cultured butter typically has a higher fat content compared to regular butter, which contributes to its rich and creamy texture.

5. Baking Delight:

Cultured butter is favored by bakers for its ability to enhance the flavor and texture of baked goods. It adds a pleasant depth to pie crusts, croissants, and cookies.

6. Bread and Pastries:

Spread it on warm bread, rolls, or toast for a delightful breakfast treat. It pairs exceptionally well with fresh artisanal bread.

7. Compound Butter:

Cultured butter can be used to create compound butter by mixing it with herbs, spices, garlic, or other flavorings. Compound butter can elevate the taste of various dishes, such as grilled steak, vegetables, or seafood.

8. Specialty Dishes:

It's a preferred choice for enhancing the flavor of gourmet dishes, from lobster bisque to pan-seared scallops.

9. Homemade Cultured Butter:

You can make cultured butter at home by allowing cream to ferment with the help of yogurt or buttermilk. The cream is then churned, and the resulting butter is strained and washed to remove any remaining buttermilk.

10. European Varieties:

European countries, particularly France, are renowned for their artisanal cultured butters, often labeled as "beurre de baratte" or "beurre fermier." These varieties are highly sought after for their exceptional quality.

Cultured butter is a delicious addition to your culinary repertoire. Its unique flavor and texture make it a gourmet choice for those seeking to enhance their cooking and baking creations. Whether you're spreading it on your morning toast, using it to finish a sauce, or incorporating it into your favorite pastry recipes, cultured butter is sure to elevate your culinary experience.

Clarified Butter: Liquid Gold

Clarified butter, known for its high smoke point and clear appearance, is a staple in many cuisines. This section will discuss how butter is clarified and its applications in cooking, particularly in Indian cuisine.

Clarified butter, often referred to as "liquid gold" in culinary circles, is a form of butter where the milk solids and water have been removed, leaving only the pure butterfat. This process has several advantages, making clarified butter highly versatile and prized in many cuisines. Here's what you need to know about clarified butter:

1. High Smoke Point:

Clarified butter has a significantly higher smoke point compared to regular butter. This means it can withstand higher cooking temperatures without burning or producing acrid smoke. Its smoke point is typically around 450°F (232°C).

2. Longer Shelf Life:

By removing the water and milk solids, clarified butter becomes more stable and less prone to spoilage. It can be stored at room temperature for extended periods without refrigeration.

3. Nutty Aroma and Flavor:

As the butterfat is heated during the clarifying process, it takes on a nutty aroma and flavor, which adds a unique and pleasant dimension to dishes.

4. Ideal for Sautéing and Frying:

The high smoke point and absence of milk solids make clarified butter an excellent choice for high-heat cooking methods like frying, sautéing, and searing.

5. Traditional in Indian Cooking:

Clarified butter, known as "ghee" in Indian cuisine, is an essential ingredient in many traditional Indian dishes. It imparts a rich, buttery flavor and is a staple in both savory and sweet recipes.

6. Perfect for Popcorn:

Many popcorn enthusiasts prefer clarified butter for drizzling over their popcorn. It offers a rich, buttery taste without the risk of burning the butter while popping.

7. Ideal for Seafood:

Clarified butter is often used for dipping or drizzling over seafood, such as lobster and crab. Its mild, nutty flavor complements the delicate taste of seafood.

8. Baking and Pastry:

While clarified butter is not typically used in baking, it can be a desirable addition to pastry recipes where a pure butterfat is needed for specific applications.

9. Homemade Clarified Butter:

You can make clarified butter at home by melting regular butter and allowing it to separate into three distinct layers: the milk solids at the bottom, the clear golden liquid (clarified butter) in the middle, and the foamy top layer. Skim off the foam and discard the milk solids to extract the clarified butter.

10. Versatile for Finishing Dishes:

Clarified butter is often used to finish dishes like vegetables, meats, and pasta. It adds a rich, buttery flavor and a glossy finish.

Clarified butter's versatility and unique qualities have earned it a revered place in many cuisines around the world. Whether you're preparing a classic Indian curry, searing a steak, or simply looking for a high-heat cooking fat with a delightful flavor, clarified butter is an excellent choice for achieving exceptional results in the kitchen.

Ghee: The Liquid Gold of India

Ghee, a revered ingredient in Indian cuisine, will be highlighted. Readers will explore the traditional method of making ghee, its importance in Indian culinary traditions, and its versatility in various dishes.

Ghee, often referred to as the "liquid gold of India," is a type of clarified butter that holds a special place in Indian cuisine and culture. It is highly prized for its unique qualities and has a rich history in the Indian subcontinent. Here's what you need to know about ghee:

1. Traditional and Sacred:

Ghee has been used in India for thousands of years and holds a sacred and cultural significance. It is often used in religious ceremonies, rituals, and offerings.

2. Nutty Aroma and Flavor:

Ghee is known for its distinct nutty aroma and rich, buttery flavor. This flavor develops during the process of simmering the butter to remove water and milk solids.

3. High Smoke Point:

Ghee has a high smoke point, typically around 450°F (232°C), making it an ideal choice for high-heat cooking methods such as frying and deep-frying.

4. Versatile Cooking Fat:

Ghee is used for a wide range of cooking applications, from sautéing and frying to roasting and grilling. It imparts a delightful flavor to dishes.

5. Lactose-Free:

The clarifying process of making ghee removes almost all the milk solids, including lactose and casein. As a result, ghee is generally well-tolerated by individuals who are lactose intolerant.

6. Longer Shelf Life:

Due to its reduced moisture content and absence of milk solids, ghee has a longer shelf life than regular butter and does not require refrigeration. It can be stored at room temperature for extended periods.

7. Nutritional Benefits:

Ghee is a source of healthy fats, including saturated fats, and is rich in fat-soluble vitamins like A, D, E, and K. It's also considered an Ayurvedic superfood with potential health benefits.

8. Culinary Applications:

Ghee is used in a wide variety of Indian dishes, from curries and dals to sweets and desserts. It's also a popular accompaniment to rice, bread, and roti.

9. Medicinal Uses:

In Ayurvedic medicine, ghee is used as a carrier for herbs and as a base for various medicinal preparations. It is believed to have healing properties.

10. Easy to Make at Home:

Ghee can be made at home by gently simmering unsalted butter to allow the water content to evaporate and the milk solids to separate and brown. The clarified liquid is then strained to produce ghee.

Ghee is cherished not only for its culinary excellence but also for its role in traditional medicine and rituals. It remains an integral part of Indian cuisine and is used in diverse ways, from adding depth to savory dishes to enhancing the sweetness of Indian desserts. Ghee's versatility and rich flavor make it a truly precious ingredient in Indian kitchens and beyond.

Cream: The Velvet Essence

The chapter will transition to cream, emphasizing its velvety texture and role in enriching dishes. Readers will learn about the types of cream, from light to heavy, and how they are used in culinary preparations.

Cream is a luxurious and versatile dairy product that is widely used in cooking and baking. It is often referred to as the "velvet essence" due to its rich and silky texture. Here's what you need to know about cream:

1. Types of Cream:

Cream comes in various forms, including heavy cream (or heavy whipping cream), light cream, half-and-half, and whipping cream. The fat content varies among these types, with heavy cream containing the most fat.

2. Fat Content:

The fat content in cream typically ranges from about 18% for light cream to 36% or more for heavy cream. The higher the fat content, the richer and thicker the cream.

3. Culinary Uses:

Cream is a key ingredient in many culinary applications. It is used to add richness and creaminess to sauces, soups, and desserts. It's often the secret to creating velvety and smooth textures in dishes.

4. Whipping Cream:

Whipping cream has a fat content that makes it suitable for whipping into stiff peaks. It's commonly used for topping desserts like pies and sundaes.

5. Thickening Agent:

Cream can be used as a thickening agent in soups and sauces. When heated, it reduces and thickens, providing body to the dish.

6. Desserts and Baking:

Cream is a vital ingredient in a wide range of desserts, from custards and ice creams to panna cotta and crème brûlée. It's also used in baking to make scones, cakes, and pastry cream.

7. Coffee and Tea:

Many people enjoy adding cream to their coffee or tea, which adds a rich and creamy element to the beverages.

8. Whipped Cream:

Whipped cream is a delightful topping for cakes, fruit, and beverages. It can be sweetened and flavored with vanilla or other extracts for added depth of flavor.

9. Savory Dishes:

Cream is a common ingredient in savory dishes like pasta sauces, gratins, and creamy soups. It balances and enhances flavors, creating a comforting and velvety mouthfeel.

10. Cream Variations:

Variations like clotted cream and crème fraîche have their unique characteristics and culinary applications. Clotted cream, for example, is a thick, spoonable cream often associated with British afternoon tea.

11. Dairy Substitutes:

For individuals who are lactose intolerant or prefer plant-based options, non-dairy cream substitutes made from ingredients like soy, almond, or coconut are available.

Cream is beloved for its ability to transform dishes into creamy, luscious creations. It's a staple in both sweet and savory cooking, adding depth, texture, and richness to a wide range of culinary creations. Whether you're indulging in a dollop of whipped cream on your dessert or using it to create a silky, luxurious sauce, cream is the embodiment of culinary decadence.

Innovations and Trends in Butter and Cream

The chapter will conclude with a look at innovations and trends in butter and cream. Readers will gain insight into contemporary approaches, such as plant-based butter and dairy-free cream alternatives, and how they cater to evolving dietary preferences.

Butter and cream, classic dairy products, have also seen their share of innovations and trends in response to changing consumer preferences and culinary advancements. Here are some innovations and trends in butter and cream:

1. Flavored Butter:

Flavored butters have gained popularity, offering a variety of options like herb-infused, garlic, truffle, or honey butter. These provide an easy way to add complexity and unique flavors to dishes.

2. Compound Butter:

Compound butters, which combine butter with herbs, spices, and other flavorings, have become more accessible. They're used for seasoning meats, vegetables, and seafood.

3. Grass-Fed and Organic:

There's a growing interest in grass-fed and organic butter. These products are considered to have higher nutritional value and offer a more sustainable and animal-friendly option.

4. Specialty Creams:

Specialty creams like crème fraîche and mascarpone have become mainstream ingredients in both savory and sweet dishes, contributing to their popularity.

5. Low-Fat and Dairy-Free Alternatives:

For those seeking lower-fat options or dairy-free alternatives, various butter and cream substitutes made from ingredients like coconut or nuts are available.

6. Artisanal and Small-Batch Production:

Artisanal butter and cream producers have gained traction, offering small-batch, handcrafted products with unique flavors and textures.

7. Whipped Cream Dispensers:

Whipped cream dispensers that use nitrous oxide cartridges have made it easier for home cooks and baristas to create freshly whipped cream with consistent results.

8. European-Style Butter:

European-style butters, with a higher fat content, have gained popularity for their richer flavor and improved baking results.

9. Grass-to-Glass:

The "grass-to-glass" trend emphasizes the connection between dairy products and the cow's diet. It's believed that the cow's diet, particularly when they graze on lush grass, can influence the flavor and nutritional profile of dairy.

10. Flavored Creams: - Flavored creams, such as vanilla, chocolate, or caramel cream, are used to add a sweet, creamy element to coffee and desserts.

11. Specialty Whipping Creams: - Specialty whipping creams with added stabilizers and flavors have become more accessible for home bakers, ensuring a consistent result for whipped cream.

12. Reduced Sodium Butter: - Innovations in butter have led to reduced sodium options, catering to those looking for lower-sodium dietary choices.

Butter and cream remain beloved ingredients in cooking and baking, and these innovations and trends reflect a growing demand for a diverse range of options to suit different tastes and dietary needs. Whether it's the creamy texture of butter, the richness of heavy cream, or the complex flavors of specialty products, butter and cream continue to play a vital role in the world of culinary creations.

Butter, Cream, and Culinary Excellence

As the chapter wraps up, readers will appreciate the role of butter and cream in elevating the culinary arts, from the simplicity of a buttered toast to the elegance of a cream-infused sauce.

Butter and cream are cornerstones of culinary excellence, cherished by chefs and home cooks alike for their ability to elevate dishes to new heights. Here's how these dairy products contribute to culinary excellence:

1. Flavor Enhancement:

Butter and cream add richness and depth of flavor to both savory and sweet dishes. Their creamy, buttery profiles enhance the taste of ingredients and create a luscious mouthfeel.

2. Texture and Creaminess:

Cream, in particular, is prized for its ability to create velvety and creamy textures. Dishes like soups, sauces, and desserts benefit from the luxurious mouthfeel that cream provides.

3. Versatility:

Butter and cream are incredibly versatile. They can be used in a wide range of recipes, from sautéing vegetables to making sauces, pastries, and decadent desserts.

4. Baking Excellence:

Butter is a fundamental ingredient in baking, where it contributes to the tenderness, flavor, and structure of baked goods like cookies, cakes, and pastries. The Maillard reaction, which occurs when butter is browned, adds complexity to baked goods.

5. Binding and Emulsifying:

Butter and cream serve as natural binders and emulsifiers in recipes. In sauces, they help stabilize emulsions and prevent separation.

6. Whipped Delights:

Whipped cream and whipped butter are essential for finishing desserts, topping beverages, and creating delightful presentations. They add elegance and visual appeal to dishes.

7. Caramelization and Browning:

Butter is a key ingredient in caramelizing onions and creating the perfect brown butter sauce. The caramelization process adds rich, nutty notes to dishes.

8. Essential for Pastries:

In pastry making, butter is used to create flaky and tender pie crusts, croissants, and puff pastry. The layering of butter in laminated doughs contributes to their signature textures.

9. Signature Dishes:

Iconic dishes like beurre blanc sauce, béarnaise sauce, and hollandaise sauce rely on butter for their distinct and luxurious flavors.

10. Custards and Ice Cream: - Cream is a key ingredient in custards and ice cream, contributing to their smooth, creamy textures and richness.

11. Balancing Spices and Heat: - Both butter and cream can help balance the heat of spicy dishes. The fats in dairy products can mitigate the intensity of chilies and other spicy ingredients.

12. Sweet and Savory Harmony: - Butter and cream seamlessly bridge the gap between sweet and savory preparations. They are equally at home in a savory pasta sauce as they are in a silky chocolate mousse.

13. Culinary Tradition: - Butter and cream have deep roots in culinary traditions worldwide. Classic French cuisine, for example, relies heavily on these dairy products to create iconic dishes.

Butter and cream are ingredients that embody culinary excellence, contributing to the creation of unforgettable flavors, textures, and experiences in the world of gastronomy. Their ability to transform ordinary ingredients into extraordinary dishes is a testament to their enduring role in culinary artistry.

CHAPTER EIGHT

Yogurt and Fermented Delights

Yogurt and other fermented dairy products have a long and celebrated history, offering a delightful combination of flavors, textures, and health benefits. In this chapter, we will explore the world of yogurt and various fermented dairy products, their production, cultural significance, and their impact on gut health.

Yogurt: The Cultured Wonder

The chapter will begin by introducing yogurt as the cultured wonder of the dairy world. Readers will learn about its unique flavor, texture, and the live bacterial cultures responsible for its transformation.

Yogurt, often described as the "cultured wonder," is a dairy product celebrated for its rich history, versatility, and health benefits. Here’s what you need to know about yogurt:

1. Fermentation Magic:

Yogurt is created through the fermentation of milk by live bacterial cultures, primarily Lactobacillus bulgaricus and Streptococcus thermophilus. This process thickens the milk and imparts its distinctive tangy flavor.

2. Ancient Origins:

Yogurt has a history dating back thousands of years, with its origins in Central Asia and the Middle East. It's believed to have been accidentally discovered by nomads who carried milk in animal-skin bags.

3. Probiotic Powerhouse:

Yogurt is a rich source of probiotics, which are beneficial bacteria that can have a positive impact on gut health. These live cultures can aid in digestion and support a balanced microbiome.

4. Nutritional Benefits:

Yogurt is packed with essential nutrients, including protein, calcium, B vitamins, and probiotics. It's often considered a nutritious addition to one's diet.

5. Versatile Ingredient:

Yogurt can be enjoyed in numerous ways, from being eaten plain or with fruit to being used in cooking, baking, and smoothies. It adds creaminess and a touch of acidity to a wide variety of dishes.

6. Greek Yogurt:

Greek yogurt is a thicker and creamier version of traditional yogurt. It's made by straining regular yogurt to remove excess whey, resulting in a higher protein content.

7. Dairy and Non-Dairy Options:

While yogurt is traditionally made from cow's milk, it's also produced from the milk of other animals like goats and sheep. Additionally, there are non-dairy alternatives made from soy, almond, coconut, and other plant-based sources.

8. Desserts and Breakfasts:

Yogurt is a popular choice for breakfast, often paired with granola, honey, or fresh fruit. It's also used in dessert recipes like parfaits and frozen yogurt.

9. Marinades and Sauces:

Yogurt's acidity and creaminess make it an excellent base for marinades, salad dressings, and sauces, such as the classic Indian dish, chicken tikka masala.

10. Beauty and Skincare: - Yogurt is used in skincare and beauty routines for its moisturizing and exfoliating properties. It's applied as a face mask or used in natural remedies.

11. Fermented Tradition: - Yogurt holds a significant place in the culinary traditions of various cultures, from Indian raita and Turkish ayran to Middle Eastern labneh.

12. Lactose Tolerance: - Some individuals with lactose intolerance can tolerate yogurt better than milk because the live cultures partially break down the lactose during fermentation.

Yogurt is a versatile and delicious addition to the world of dairy products. Whether you savor it on its own, incorporate it into cooking, or benefit from its probiotic properties, yogurt continues to be a cultured wonder with a rich history and a promising future.

Yogurt Making: Bacterial Alchemy

Readers will journey through the fascinating process of yogurt making. They will understand how bacterial cultures, such as Lactobacillus and

Streptococcus, ferment milk to produce the creamy and tangy delight that is yogurt.

Yogurt making is a fascinating process of bacterial alchemy that transforms milk into a creamy and tangy dairy delight. Here's how yogurt is made:

1. Ingredients:

The primary ingredient for yogurt making is milk, which can be from various sources, including cow, goat, sheep, or plant-based alternatives like soy or coconut milk. Additionally, you'll need a small amount of yogurt with live active cultures to serve as a starter.

2. Heating:

The first step involves heating the milk to a specific temperature, typically around 180°F (82°C). This heat treatment serves several purposes, including pasteurizing the milk to kill any harmful bacteria and denaturing the milk proteins to promote thickening.

3. Cooling:

After heating, the milk is cooled to a temperature of around 110-115°F (43-46°C). This is the ideal range for the live bacterial cultures to thrive and ferment the milk.

4. Inoculation:

A small amount of the live yogurt culture is mixed into the warm milk. The live cultures typically include Lactobacillus bulgaricus and Streptococcus thermophilus, but other strains may be added for specific yogurt varieties.

5. Fermentation:

The inoculated milk is left to ferment for several hours, usually between 4 to 12 hours, at a controlled temperature. During this time, the live cultures convert lactose (milk sugar) into lactic acid, which thickens the milk and imparts the characteristic tangy flavor of yogurt.

6. Thickening and Setting:

As the fermentation progresses, the milk thickens and sets into a custard-like consistency. The longer the fermentation, the tangier and thicker the yogurt will become.

7. Cooling and Storage:

Once the yogurt has reached the desired consistency and flavor, it is cooled and then refrigerated. Cooling stops the fermentation process. The yogurt can be consumed immediately or stored in the refrigerator for later use.

8. Flavoring and Additions:

At this point, you can enjoy the yogurt as is, or you can flavor it with sweeteners, fruits, honey, or spices, depending on your preference. You can also add granola or nuts for extra texture.

9. Straining (Optional):

Greek yogurt is made by straining regular yogurt to remove excess whey, resulting in a thicker, creamier product. This step is optional and can be done by placing the yogurt in a cheesecloth or muslin bag and allowing the whey to drain off.

10. Reusing as a Starter: - You can reserve a portion of the freshly made yogurt to use as a starter for your next batch. This way, you can continue making yogurt without having to purchase commercial yogurt each time.

Yogurt making is a simple yet magical process that highlights the transformative power of beneficial bacteria. Whether you enjoy it plain or with various toppings, homemade yogurt allows you to customize the flavor and texture to your liking while reaping the probiotic benefits of live cultures.

Types of Yogurt

The chapter will explore the diverse world of yogurt varieties, from plain and Greek yogurt to fruit-flavored and probiotic-rich options. Readers will learn how different types of yogurt cater to various tastes and dietary preferences.

Yogurt comes in a variety of types and styles, each offering its unique characteristics and flavors. Here are some of the most common types of yogurt:

1. Plain Yogurt:

This is the most basic type of yogurt, made from just milk and live bacterial cultures. It has a tangy flavor and can vary in texture from creamy to somewhat thin.

2. Greek Yogurt:

Greek yogurt is known for its thick and creamy consistency. It's made by straining regular yogurt to remove excess whey, resulting in a higher protein content. Greek yogurt is versatile and is used in both sweet and savory dishes.

3. Regular (Full-Fat) Yogurt:

Full-fat yogurt is made with whole milk and contains a higher fat content. It has a rich, creamy texture and is known for its satisfying mouthfeel.

4. Low-Fat Yogurt:

Low-fat yogurt is made with reduced-fat milk, making it a lighter option while still providing the benefits of yogurt. It has a lower fat content than full-fat yogurt.

5. Fat-Free (Non-Fat) Yogurt:

Fat-free yogurt is made from skim milk, containing little to no fat. It's a popular choice for those seeking a lower-calorie option.

6. Flavored Yogurt:

Flavored yogurts have added sweeteners, fruit purees, or flavorings to enhance the taste. Popular flavors include vanilla, strawberry, blueberry, and more.

7. Fruit on the Bottom:

This style of yogurt features fruit preserves or compotes at the bottom of the container. It allows you to mix the fruit into the yogurt as desired.

8. Drinkable Yogurt (Yogurt Smoothie):

Drinkable yogurt is a liquid form of yogurt, often sweetened and flavored. It's convenient for on-the-go consumption.

9. Skyr:

Skyr is an Icelandic yogurt known for its thick, creamy texture and high protein content. It's similar to Greek yogurt and is traditionally made with specific bacterial cultures.

10. Kefir: - Kefir is a fermented dairy product that's thinner and more drinkable than traditional yogurt. It contains a diverse range of probiotic bacteria and yeast cultures.

11. Labneh: - Labneh is a strained yogurt with a thick, spreadable consistency. It's often used in Middle Eastern and Mediterranean cuisines and can be flavored with herbs and spices.

12. Plant-Based Yogurt: - Plant-based yogurt is a dairy-free alternative made from sources like soy, almond, coconut, or cashews. It offers options for those with dairy allergies or dietary preferences.

13. Lactose-Free Yogurt: - Lactose-free yogurt is made for individuals who are lactose intolerant. It contains the same live bacterial cultures but with the lactose pre-digested.

14. Probiotic Yogurt: - Probiotic yogurt contains additional live probiotic cultures that are believed to provide extra digestive health benefits.

15. Child-Friendly Yogurt: - These yogurts are often marketed towards children and come in kid-friendly flavors and packaging. They may also contain added vitamins and minerals.

Each type of yogurt has its own flavor, texture, and nutritional profile, allowing you to choose the one that best suits your taste preferences and dietary needs. Whether you prefer the tang of plain yogurt, the creaminess of Greek yogurt, or the convenience of drinkable yogurt, there's a yogurt variety for everyone.

Kefir: The Fermented Elixir

The chapter will introduce kefir, a fermented dairy product known for its effervescence and unique probiotic profile. Readers will explore the fermentation process and the significance of kefir in various cultures.

Kefir is often referred to as a "fermented elixir" due to its unique characteristics and potential health benefits. Here's a closer look at kefir:

1. Fermentation Process:

Kefir is made by fermenting milk with kefir grains, which are a combination of live bacterial cultures and yeast. This combination of microorganisms gives kefir its distinctive properties.

2. Origins:

Kefir has its roots in the Caucasus Mountains, where it has been made for centuries. It's believed to have been a gift from the gods because of its remarkable health benefits.

3. Probiotic Powerhouse:

Kefir is a potent source of probiotics, containing a wide variety of beneficial bacteria and yeast strains. These probiotics can have a positive impact on gut health, aiding digestion and supporting the balance of the microbiome.

4. Thick and Creamy Texture:

Kefir has a creamy consistency that falls somewhere between liquid yogurt and a smoothie. Its thickness can vary based on the fermentation time and temperature.

5. Tangy Flavor:

Kefir has a tart and slightly tangy flavor, which can be milder or more pronounced, depending on factors such as fermentation time and temperature.

6. Dairy and Non-Dairy Varieties:

While traditional kefir is made from cow's or goat's milk, non-dairy alternatives are also available, using bases like coconut milk, soy milk, or almond milk.

7. Fermentation Time:

Kefir is typically fermented for 12 to 24 hours, which is longer than the fermentation process for regular yogurt. This extended fermentation time contributes to its unique microbial composition.

8. Effervescence:

Due to the carbon dioxide produced during fermentation, kefir can have a slight effervescence or fizziness, giving it a refreshing quality.

9. Versatile Use:

Kefir can be enjoyed on its own or used in a variety of culinary applications. It's commonly used in smoothies, salad dressings, marinades, or as a base for soups and dips.

10. Nutritional Profile: - Kefir is rich in nutrients, including protein, calcium, B vitamins, and beneficial probiotics. It's often considered a nutrient-dense food.

11. Lactose Tolerance: - Some people with lactose intolerance can tolerate kefir better than milk

because the live cultures in kefir partially digest the lactose.

12. Potential Health Benefits: - Kefir is associated with various health benefits, such as improved gut health, enhanced immunity, and potential anti-inflammatory properties. However, more research is needed to fully understand these effects.

13. Home Fermentation: - Kefir can be made at home using kefir grains, which can be reused for multiple batches. This makes it a cost-effective way to enjoy homemade probiotic-rich kefir.

Kefir's unique combination of probiotics and its distinct flavor and texture have made it a popular fermented dairy product around the world. It's not only appreciated for its potential health benefits but also for its culinary versatility and refreshing taste.

Yogurt, Fermented Delights, and Health

As the chapter wraps up, readers will recognize the connection between yogurt and fermented dairy products and potential health benefits, from digestive health to immune support, and how these products continue to find their place in contemporary diets.

Yogurt and other fermented delights are not only delicious but also have potential health benefits due to their probiotic content and other nutritional qualities. Here's an overview of how these foods can contribute to well-being:

1. Probiotic Power:

Fermented foods like yogurt, kefir, sauerkraut, kimchi, and miso are rich in probiotics, which are beneficial bacteria that support gut health. Consuming probiotics can help maintain a balanced gut microbiome, which is essential for digestion, nutrient absorption, and immune function.

2. Improved Digestion:

Probiotics in fermented foods can aid digestion by promoting the breakdown of food and the absorption of nutrients. They may also alleviate common digestive issues, such as diarrhea, constipation, and irritable bowel syndrome (IBS).

3. Enhanced Immunity:

A healthy gut is closely linked to a strong immune system. Regular consumption of probiotic-rich foods can help boost the body's defense mechanisms against infections and illnesses.

4. Lactose Tolerance:

For individuals with lactose intolerance, yogurt and kefir may be better tolerated than regular milk due to the enzymatic action of probiotics that partially digest lactose. This can make dairy more accessible for those with lactose sensitivity.

5. Nutrient Density:

Fermented foods are nutrient-dense, containing vitamins, minerals, and other essential nutrients. Yogurt, for example, is a good source of calcium, protein, and B vitamins.

6. Weight Management:

Some research suggests that probiotics from fermented foods may assist in weight management by supporting a healthy metabolism and reducing inflammation.

7. Mental Health:

Emerging research is exploring the connection between gut health and mental health. The gut-brain axis suggests that a healthy gut microbiome may have a positive influence on mood and cognitive function.

8. Heart Health:

The probiotics in fermented foods may contribute to heart health by helping to regulate blood pressure and reduce cholesterol levels. Additionally, yogurt is a source of potassium, which can support heart function.

9. Bone Health:

Dairy-based fermented foods, like yogurt, provide calcium and vitamin D, both crucial for bone health and the prevention of osteoporosis.

10. Reduced Inflammation: - Chronic inflammation is linked to various health problems. Some studies suggest that probiotics in fermented foods may help reduce systemic inflammation.

11. Allergen Tolerance: - Early exposure to probiotics from fermented foods might contribute to the development of a well-balanced immune system and lower the risk of allergies and asthma in children.

12. Skin Health: - A healthy gut may contribute to better skin health. Some individuals report improvements in skin conditions like acne, eczema, and psoriasis when they consume probiotics regularly.

13. Longevity: - There is ongoing research into whether a balanced gut microbiome, influenced by

probiotics, could have an impact on longevity and age-related diseases.

It's important to note that while fermented foods have potential health benefits, individual responses can vary, and not all fermented foods are equal in terms of probiotic content. Choosing products with live active cultures and a wide variety of probiotic strains can be particularly beneficial.

Additionally, the overall diet and lifestyle, including exercise, stress management, and sleep, play a significant role in one's health and well-being. Fermented foods can be a valuable component of a balanced and health-supportive diet.

CHAPTER NINE

Dairy and Human Health

The relationship between dairy products and human health is a complex and multifaceted one. In this chapter, we will delve into the scientific evidence surrounding the impact of dairy consumption on various aspects of human health, including bone health, cardiovascular health, weight management, and more.

Dairy and Dental Health

The role of dairy in dental health will be explored. Readers will understand how the calcium and phosphorus in dairy help maintain healthy teeth, preventing tooth decay and gum disease.

The relationship between dairy consumption and dental health is an important aspect of overall well-being. Here's an overview of how dairy can positively impact dental health:

1. Calcium and Phosphorus:

Dairy products are rich in calcium and phosphorus, which are essential minerals for maintaining strong teeth. These minerals play a crucial role in the remineralization of tooth enamel and preventing tooth decay.

2. Casein Protein:

Dairy contains casein, a protein that forms a protective film on the surface of teeth. This film can help prevent harmful acids and bacteria from eroding tooth enamel.

3. Reduction of Acidity:

Dairy products, particularly milk, can help neutralize the acids in the mouth that are produced by harmful bacteria. This reduction in acidity can lower the risk of tooth decay.

4. Cheese's Protective Properties:

Cheese, in particular, has been found to have protective properties for dental health. It can stimulate saliva production, which helps to wash away food particles and harmful acids, and it provides a source of calcium and phosphorus.

5. Probiotics in Yogurt:

Some dairy products like yogurt contain probiotics, which can contribute to a balanced oral microbiome. A balanced oral microbiome can help prevent the growth of harmful bacteria that lead to cavities and gum disease.

It's important to note that while dairy can be beneficial for dental health, there are factors to consider:

1. Added Sugars:

Some flavored dairy products, such as sweetened yogurt and flavored milk, can contain added sugars that may contribute to tooth decay if consumed in excess. Choosing unsweetened or plain dairy products is a better option for dental health.

2. Lactose Intolerance:

Some individuals may be lactose intolerant, and consuming dairy products could lead to gastrointestinal discomfort. In such cases, lactose-free dairy or non-dairy alternatives can be suitable choices.

3. Dental Hygiene:

Good dental hygiene practices, including regular brushing, flossing, and dental check-ups, are essential for maintaining dental health, and dairy should be considered as part of an overall dental care routine.

In conclusion, dairy products, especially when consumed in their natural form without added sugars, can play a positive role in maintaining dental health. The combination of calcium, phosphorus, and protective proteins in dairy can help protect tooth enamel and prevent tooth decay. However, it's important to practice good dental hygiene and consider individual dietary preferences and sensitivities when incorporating dairy into one's diet.

Dairy and Cardiovascular Health

The chapter will examine the relationship between dairy consumption and cardiovascular health. Readers will gain insight into the impact of saturated fats in dairy and the potential benefits of consuming low-fat and non-fat dairy products for heart health.

The relationship between dairy consumption and cardiovascular health is an important topic in nutrition and health research. Here's an overview of the impact of dairy on cardiovascular health:

1. Saturated Fats:

Dairy products, especially full-fat varieties like whole milk and cheese, can be significant sources of saturated fats. High intake of saturated fats has traditionally been associated with an increased risk of cardiovascular diseases, such as heart disease and stroke.

2. Low-Fat and Non-Fat Options:

Many dairy products offer low-fat and non-fat alternatives. These options reduce the saturated fat content, making them more heart-healthy choices.

3. Nutrient Content:

Dairy products, even those with some saturated fats, provide essential nutrients like calcium, vitamin D, and protein. These nutrients are crucial for overall health, and they can be obtained from dairy without excessive saturated fat intake.

4. Calcium and Blood Pressure:

Some research suggests that a diet rich in calcium, which is abundant in dairy products, may have a modest lowering effect on blood pressure, potentially reducing the risk of hypertension and related cardiovascular issues.

5. Dairy and the Mediterranean Diet:

In Mediterranean-style diets, which emphasize a variety of nutrient-rich foods, moderate dairy consumption is part of a heart-healthy eating pattern.

6. Fermented Dairy and Probiotics:

Some dairy products like yogurt and kefir contain probiotics, which can contribute to gut health. An unhealthy gut microbiome has been linked to an increased risk of cardiovascular diseases.

7. Individual Variation:

The impact of dairy on cardiovascular health can vary from person to person. Genetics, overall diet, and lifestyle factors play a role in how dairy consumption affects an individual's heart health.

8. Moderation and Balance:

The key to incorporating dairy into a heart-healthy diet is moderation and balance. Opting for low-fat or non-fat dairy options and balancing dairy with other nutrient-rich foods like fruits, vegetables, and whole grains can help reduce the potential negative effects of saturated fats.

It's important to note that current dietary guidelines recommend moderation in saturated fat intake, and individuals with specific cardiovascular risk factors or dietary preferences may choose to limit their saturated fat intake from dairy sources. Overall, dairy can be a part of a heart-healthy diet when chosen wisely and consumed as part of a balanced and varied diet. Individuals should consider their unique dietary needs and consult with healthcare professionals or nutritionists when making dietary choices related to cardiovascular health.

Dairy and Mental Health

The chapter will also examine emerging research on the potential impact of dairy on mental health. Readers will explore the relationship between dairy nutrients and conditions like depression and anxiety.

The relationship between dairy consumption and mental health is a topic of emerging research and interest. While it's an area that continues to be explored, here's an overview of the potential impact of dairy on mental health:

1. Nutrient Content:

Dairy products are rich in essential nutrients, including vitamins, minerals, and proteins, which are known to support overall health. Some of these nutrients, such as B vitamins and vitamin D, play a role in brain health and function.

2. Vitamin D and Mental Health:

Vitamin D, which is naturally present in some dairy products and fortified in others, has been associated with mood regulation. Low levels of vitamin D have been linked to conditions like depression, and adequate vitamin D intake may have a positive impact on mental well-being.

3. Omega-3 Fatty Acids:

Some dairy products, like certain types of cheese, contain omega-3 fatty acids. Omega-3s have been studied for their potential to reduce the risk of mood disorders and improve cognitive function.

4. Probiotics and the Gut-Brain Connection:

Probiotic-rich dairy products, such as yogurt, may influence the gut microbiome, which is increasingly recognized for its role in the gut-brain axis. A balanced gut microbiome is believed to have a positive influence on mood and mental health.

5. Protein for Brain Function:

Dairy is a source of high-quality protein, which is essential for brain function. Protein provides the amino acids needed for the production of neurotransmitters, which play a role in mood and cognition.

6. Dairy and Inflammation:

Chronic inflammation has been linked to various mental health conditions. Some research suggests that dairy products may help control inflammation, potentially benefiting mental health.

It's important to note that while there are potential benefits, the impact of dairy on mental health is highly individual. Some individuals may be sensitive to dairy or lactose intolerant, and for them, dairy consumption could have adverse effects on digestion and overall well-being.

A well-rounded diet that includes a variety of nutrient-rich foods, along with other factors like regular physical activity, stress management, and social support, plays a significant role in mental health. As research in this area continues, a balanced perspective on the relationship between dairy and mental well-being is essential, and individuals should make dietary choices that align with their unique needs and preferences.

Dairy and Immune Health

The impact of dairy on the immune system will be discussed. Readers will gain insight into the potential role of probiotic-rich dairy products in supporting immune function.

The potential impact of dairy on immune health is an area of growing interest and research. Here's an overview of the connection between dairy, probiotics, and the immune system:

1. Probiotic-Rich Dairy Products:

Some dairy products, like yogurt and kefir, are rich in probiotics, which are live beneficial bacteria that can positively influence the gut microbiome. A balanced gut microbiome is closely linked to a well-functioning immune system.

2. Gut-Immune Connection:

The gut is a significant player in immune function. The majority of immune cells reside in the gut-associated lymphoid tissue (GALT). A healthy gut microbiome, influenced by probiotics, can help regulate immune responses.

3. Immune Modulation:

Probiotics in dairy may help modulate the immune system by promoting the production of antibodies and cytokines. This can enhance the body's defense against infections and diseases.

4. Respiratory Infections:

Some studies suggest that probiotics from dairy products might reduce the risk and severity of respiratory infections, such as the common cold and flu.

5. Allergic Reactions:

Probiotics in dairy may play a role in reducing the risk of allergies and allergic reactions by helping to balance immune responses.

6. Gut-Brain Connection:

Emerging research explores the gut-brain axis, which suggests that a healthy gut influenced by probiotics could have a positive impact on mood, stress responses, and mental health.

7. Inflammation Control:

Chronic inflammation is linked to numerous health issues. A balanced gut microbiome supported by probiotics may help control systemic inflammation, reducing the risk of inflammatory diseases.

8. Immune System Support:

Probiotics from dairy may help the immune system differentiate between harmful pathogens and harmless substances, preventing inappropriate immune responses as seen in autoimmune conditions.

It's essential to note that the specific strains of probiotics, their dosage, and the overall diet and lifestyle all play a crucial role in their impact on immune health. Not all dairy products contain probiotics, so selecting those labeled with live active cultures is important.

While probiotic-rich dairy products can be a valuable part of a diet that supports immune health, a well-rounded diet, regular physical activity, and overall lifestyle factors also contribute significantly to a robust immune system. As research in this field continues to evolve, a balanced perspective on dairy's role in immune health is essential.

CHAPTER TEN

Milk Beyond the Glass

Milk is not just a beverage but a versatile ingredient that plays a crucial role in the world of culinary arts. In this chapter, we will explore the myriad ways in which milk is used as a foundational ingredient in various dairy products and dishes, enriching the culinary landscape.

Milk as a Kitchen Staple

The chapter will commence by highlighting the ubiquitous presence of milk in kitchens worldwide. Readers will learn how milk serves as a foundational ingredient, contributing to the textures, flavors, and consistency of countless recipes.

Milk is a versatile and essential kitchen staple used in a wide range of culinary applications. Here are some of the common ways milk is used in the kitchen:

Baking: Milk is a key ingredient in many baking recipes. It adds moisture, tenderness, and richness to baked goods like cakes, cookies, muffins, and bread.

Sauces and Gravies: Milk is often used as a base for creamy sauces and gravies, such as béchamel and alfredo sauce. It helps thicken the sauce and adds a creamy texture.

Cereal and Oatmeal: Milk is a classic choice for pouring over breakfast cereals and oatmeal. It adds a creamy and slightly sweet element to these morning staples.

Hot Drinks: Milk is commonly used in hot drinks like coffee, tea, and hot chocolate. It can be frothed or steamed for cappuccinos and lattes.

Smoothies: Milk is a popular choice as the liquid base for smoothies. It adds creaminess and a source of nutrients to blended drinks.

Mashed Potatoes: Some people use milk to make creamy mashed potatoes. It helps achieve a smooth and fluffy texture.

Scrambled Eggs: A splash of milk can be added to scrambled eggs to make them fluffier and lighter.

Desserts: Milk is a primary ingredient in various dessert recipes, including custards, puddings, and ice creams. It contributes to the smooth and creamy texture of these sweets.

Soups: Milk is used in some creamy soups, such as clam chowder or corn chowder, to create a rich and velvety consistency.

Marinades: Milk can be used in marinades for meats, particularly in some Southern fried chicken recipes. It helps tenderize and flavor the meat.

Pasta Dishes: Milk can be used in pasta dishes to create creamy sauces, such as fettuccine alfredo or macaroni and cheese.

Doughs: In some bread and pastry recipes, milk is an ingredient that can improve the texture and flavor of the dough.

Custard-Based Dishes: Milk is a key component in custard-based dishes like quiches and flans.

Casseroles: Some casserole recipes call for milk to bind the ingredients and create a creamy texture.

Milkshakes: Milk serves as the base for milkshakes, blended with ice cream and flavorings to create a delicious, creamy beverage.

When using milk in cooking, it's important to choose the right type of milk for the recipe. Whole milk, 2% milk, and skim milk can be used in different dishes depending on the desired fat content. Additionally, lactose-free and plant-based milk alternatives are available for those with dietary restrictions or preferences.

The Magic of Milk in Baking

Readers will delve into the role of milk in baking, from its use in creating tender and moist cakes to the essential component of bread-making. This section will explore the science of milk's interaction with leavening agents and gluten.

Milk plays a magical role in baking, contributing to the texture, flavor, and overall quality of a wide range of baked goods. Here's how milk works its magic in baking:

1. Moisture: Milk is an excellent source of moisture in baking. It provides hydration to the flour and

other dry ingredients, which is essential for gluten development. This hydration helps create a tender and moist crumb in cakes, muffins, and bread.

2. Fat: Depending on the type of milk used (whole, 2%, skim, or buttermilk), milk contributes varying amounts of fat to baked goods. Fat adds richness, tenderness, and flavor to the final product. Whole milk and buttermilk, with their higher fat content, result in a more tender and flavorful crumb.

3. Binding: Milk contains proteins that act as binders in baking. These proteins help hold the ingredients together and provide structure to baked goods.

4. Flavor: Milk has a mild, slightly sweet flavor that can enhance the taste of baked goods. It complements the sweetness of sugar and the richness of butter, resulting in a balanced flavor profile.

5. Color: Milk can contribute to the browning of baked goods. This is particularly evident in recipes like bread and rolls, where the proteins and sugars in milk participate in the Maillard reaction, creating a golden crust.

6. Leavening: In some recipes, milk can serve as a leavening agent when combined with baking soda

or baking powder. This combination produces carbon dioxide gas, which helps baked goods rise and become light and airy.

7. Creaminess: In custards, puddings, and creamy fillings, milk is a primary ingredient that provides a smooth, creamy, and luscious texture. It's the foundation for creating the perfect custard or pudding.

8. Balance: Milk can balance the acidity in recipes that include acidic ingredients like buttermilk or sour cream. This balance can result in a more even rise and better texture in baked goods.

9. Versatility: Milk is a versatile ingredient that can be used in a variety of baked goods, from sweet to savory. It can be added to cookies, cakes, quick breads, pancakes, waffles, quiches, and more.

When using milk in baking, it's important to choose the type of milk that best suits the recipe. Whole milk adds richness, while lower-fat options like 2% or skim milk provide moisture without the extra fat. Buttermilk is often used in recipes for its tangy flavor and leavening properties.

In summary, milk is a baking staple that contributes to the structure, texture, flavor, and overall quality of a wide array of baked goods. Its moisture, fat, and binding properties make it an essential ingredient for creating delicious treats in the kitchen.

Creamy Sauces and Gravies

Milk forms the base for a multitude of creamy sauces and gravies in cuisines around the world. Readers will understand how milk enriches the flavors and textures of dishes like béchamel sauce and sausage gravy.

Creamy sauces and gravies are beloved for their rich, velvety texture and decadent flavor. They are versatile and can be used in a variety of savory dishes to add a creamy element. Here's how to make creamy sauces and gravies:

Ingredients:

2 tablespoons of butter or a neutral cooking oil

2 tablespoons of all-purpose flour

1 cup of milk (whole milk or half-and-half for creamier results)

Salt and pepper to taste

Optional seasonings such as garlic, onion, herbs, or spices

Instructions:

Melt the Fat: In a saucepan over medium heat, melt the butter (or heat the cooking oil) until it's sizzling. You can also add minced garlic or diced onions at this stage for added flavor.

Add the Flour: Sprinkle the flour over the melted fat and whisk continuously to create a smooth paste. This mixture is called a roux, and it will thicken the sauce.

Cook the Roux: Keep stirring the roux for about 1-2 minutes, ensuring it doesn't brown. Cooking the roux helps eliminate the raw taste of the flour.

Gradually Add Milk: Slowly pour in the milk while whisking constantly. Adding the milk gradually prevents lumps from forming. Continue to whisk until the mixture is smooth.

Simmer and Thicken: Bring the sauce to a gentle simmer over medium heat, still whisking. As it simmers, the sauce will thicken. This can take about 5-7 minutes. If it thickens too much, you can add more milk to reach your desired consistency.

Season: Season the sauce with salt, pepper, and any additional seasonings or spices to taste. Taste the sauce and adjust the seasoning as needed.

Serve: Once the sauce has reached the desired thickness and is well-seasoned, remove it from the heat. It's now ready to be poured over your dish.

Variations:

Cheese Sauce: To make a cheese sauce, add shredded cheese (such as cheddar, parmesan, or gruyere) to the sauce and stir until it's fully melted and smooth.

Creamy Gravy: To make a creamy gravy for dishes like biscuits and gravy, use chicken or turkey broth in place of milk and season with salt, pepper, and herbs.

Mushroom Sauce: Sauté sliced mushrooms in the butter before adding flour. Once they are tender, proceed with the recipe as usual.

Creamy sauces and gravies can be used on a variety of dishes, from pasta and vegetables to mashed potatoes and meat. They add a luxurious and comforting element to many recipes, making them a favorite in both home cooking and restaurant cuisine.

Milk and the Art of Puddings and Custards

Readers will explore the art of puddings and custards, where milk is a fundamental ingredient.

This section will provide an understanding of the science behind custard formation and the versatility of dairy in creating a wide range of sweet and savory puddings.

Milk is a fundamental ingredient in the creation of puddings and custards, two classic and beloved dessert categories. Here’s how milk contributes to the art of making these delectable treats:

Puddings:

Creamy Texture: Milk is the primary liquid used in pudding recipes, whether it’s a stovetop or baked pudding. The milk contributes to the creamy and smooth texture that is characteristic of puddings.

Flavor Enhancement: Milk has a mild and slightly sweet flavor that complements the other ingredients in the pudding, such as sugar, vanilla, and chocolate. It enhances the overall taste of the dessert.

Gelatinization: Puddings are thickened with starch, typically cornstarch, and the gelatinization process is crucial for achieving the right consistency. Milk plays a vital role in this process, helping the starch granules absorb liquid and swell to create a thickened, pudding-like texture.

Setting Agent: When the pudding is cooled, it firms up and sets, forming a custard-like consistency. The proteins in milk contribute to this setting process, helping the pudding maintain its shape.

Versatility: Milk-based puddings can be flavored in countless ways, from classic vanilla to chocolate, butterscotch, and fruit flavors. Milk provides a neutral canvas for various flavorings.

Custards:

Creaminess: Custards, whether they are baked or stovetop versions, rely on milk (and often cream) for their creamy and velvety texture. The milk contributes to the luxurious mouthfeel of custards.

Setting and Binding: In custards, eggs are the primary thickening and setting agents. Milk acts as the liquid medium that combines with eggs to create a smooth and custardy consistency when cooked.

Flavor Balance: Milk's mild and slightly sweet flavor balances the richness of egg yolks and any added flavorings, such as vanilla or nutmeg. This balance is essential for achieving a well-rounded taste.

Uniform Heating: The high water content of milk helps distribute heat evenly during the cooking process, ensuring that the custard cooks at a steady rate without curdling or separating.

Versatility: Custards can be flavored in various ways, allowing for a wide range of desserts, from classic crème brûlée to flan, quiches, and ice creams.

Milk in Coffee and Tea

Milk is a beloved addition to coffee and tea, and this section will highlight its role in creating the perfect cup. Readers will learn about the various types of milk used for frothing and steaming, enhancing the aroma and flavor of these beloved beverages.

Milk is a popular and versatile addition to coffee and tea, enhancing flavor, texture, and overall enjoyment. Here's how milk is used in these beloved beverages:

In Coffee:

Texture and Creaminess: Milk adds a creamy and velvety texture to coffee, which can counterbalance the bitterness or acidity of some coffee types. This creaminess can make the coffee smoother and more enjoyable to drink.

Taste Balance: The mild sweetness of milk can balance the flavor of coffee, especially in dark or strong brews. It can mellow out the coffee's intensity and make it more approachable for a wider range of palates.

Temperature Adjustment: Milk can be heated before adding it to coffee, allowing you to control the temperature of your beverage. Whether you prefer your coffee piping hot or just warm, milk can help achieve the desired temperature.

Foam and Froth: Milk is a key component in creating foam and froth for espresso-based drinks like cappuccinos and lattes. Steamed milk is frothed to create the creamy, velvety topping that's a signature of these beverages.

Customization: The choice of milk can vary from person to person. Some prefer whole milk for its richness, while others opt for skim or non-dairy alternatives like almond or soy milk to suit dietary preferences.

In Tea:

Creaminess: Milk can add a creamy element to tea, particularly black tea varieties. It softens the astringency and adds a pleasant, rounded mouthfeel.

Balancing Tannins: Tea contains tannins, which can contribute to a slightly bitter or astringent taste. Milk can help neutralize these tannins and create a smoother tea-drinking experience.

Variation in Tea Types: While milk is commonly added to black teas, it can also be used with chai, matcha lattes, and herbal teas, each contributing a unique flavor and texture to the beverage.

Cultural Variations: The way milk is added to tea varies by culture. In British tradition, milk is added after the tea is poured, while in Indian chai, it is often simmered with the tea and spices. Thai tea and Hong Kong-style milk tea are other examples of milk-infused teas.

Sweetening: Some tea drinkers add sugar along with milk to create a sweet, creamy tea. This is particularly common in masala chai and Thai tea.

Milk in Ethnic Cuisines

The chapter will showcase how milk is used in diverse ethnic cuisines, from the creamy curries of

Indian cuisine to the milk-based desserts of Middle Eastern and South Asian cultures. Readers will gain an appreciation for the unique flavor profiles created by dairy.

Milk plays a significant role in a wide range of ethnic cuisines around the world. Its versatility makes it a staple ingredient in both savory and sweet dishes. Here's a look at how milk is used in various ethnic cuisines:

Indian Cuisine:

Chai: India is famous for its spiced tea, known as chai. Milk is an essential component of chai, creating a creamy and aromatic beverage when combined with black tea, spices (such as cardamom, cinnamon, and cloves), and sugar.

Paneer: Paneer is a fresh cheese made by curdling milk with an acid like lemon juice or vinegar. It's a key ingredient in Indian dishes like palak paneer and paneer tikka.

Kheer: Kheer is a sweet rice pudding made with milk, rice, sugar, and aromatic ingredients like cardamom and saffron.

Italian Cuisine:

Risotto: Milk is often used to make creamy risotto, a popular Italian dish. It's added gradually to rice to create a rich, velvety texture.

Tiramisu: Tiramisu is a classic Italian dessert that features mascarpone cheese, which is made from cream. It's combined with espresso-soaked ladyfingers and dusted with cocoa powder.

Alfredo Sauce: Alfredo sauce, a creamy pasta sauce, typically includes butter, heavy cream, and Parmesan cheese.

Mexican Cuisine:

Horchata: Horchata is a sweet, rice-based beverage flavored with cinnamon and vanilla. Milk or condensed milk is often used in the preparation of horchata.

Tres Leches Cake: This popular Mexican dessert features a sponge cake soaked in a mixture of three milks: evaporated milk, condensed milk, and whole milk.

Thai Cuisine:

Tom Kha Gai: This classic Thai soup features coconut milk, chicken, and an assortment of aromatic herbs and spices. The coconut milk adds a creamy and slightly sweet element to the dish.

Thai Iced Tea: Thai iced tea is a sweet and creamy beverage made from brewed black tea, sweetened condensed milk, and evaporated milk. It's often served over ice.

Middle Eastern Cuisine:

Rice Pudding: Middle Eastern cuisine is known for its creamy and fragrant rice pudding, flavored with rosewater or orange blossom water.

Muhallebi: Muhallebi is a popular milk-based dessert made with milk, sugar, and rice or cornstarch. It's typically garnished with pistachios or other nuts.

Scandinavian Cuisine:

Swedish Meatballs: Swedish meatballs are often served with a creamy sauce made from beef broth, heavy cream, and sometimes milk. This sauce is a key component of the dish.

Rice Porridge: Rice porridge, often consumed on Christmas morning, is made by simmering rice with milk and is sweetened with cinnamon and sugar.

Chinese Cuisine:

Congee: Chinese congee, a rice porridge, is often made with a mixture of rice and water, but milk can be used to create a creamier variation. It can be sweet or savory and served with various toppings.

Milk's contribution to these cuisines varies from enhancing texture to providing creaminess and a touch of sweetness. It plays a key role in creating a wide array of delightful dishes and beverages enjoyed by people around the world.

Milk and Sweets

Readers will explore the world of sweet delights where milk plays a central role. From ice creams to truffles, they will understand how milk enriches the texture and flavor of various confections.

Milk is a fundamental ingredient in the world of sweets, contributing to the creaminess, richness, and flavor of a wide range of desserts. Here's how milk is used in sweet treats:

Ice Cream: Milk is one of the primary components of ice cream, along with cream, sugar, and flavorings. It provides the smooth and creamy texture of ice cream. Variations like gelato and sorbet also use milk, albeit in different proportions.

Puddings: Milk is the key ingredient in various pudding recipes, including rice pudding, bread pudding, and tapioca pudding. It's heated with sugar and starch to create a thick and creamy dessert.

Custards: Custard desserts, like crème brûlée and flan, rely on milk for their smooth and silky texture. Eggs are often added to create a firm yet delicate consistency.

Chocolate: Milk chocolate is made by adding milk powder or condensed milk to cocoa mass and sugar. This results in a sweet and creamy chocolate that's a favorite for candy bars and baking.

Cakes: Milk is a common component in cake recipes, contributing to the moistness and flavor of the cake. It's often used in conjunction with other dairy products like butter or cream.

Tres Leches Cake: As mentioned earlier, this Latin American dessert involves soaking a sponge cake in a mixture of three milks: evaporated milk, condensed milk, and whole milk. The result is a luscious and moist cake.

Hot Chocolate: A comforting and sweet beverage, hot chocolate combines milk with cocoa powder or chocolate bars, sugar, and sometimes a touch of cream. It's often garnished with whipped cream or marshmallows.

Milkshakes: A classic milkshake consists of milk, ice cream, and flavorings like chocolate syrup, fruit, or vanilla extract. It's blended into a thick, sweet, and indulgent drink.

Caramel: Caramel candies and sauces are created by heating sugar and milk or cream together. The milk contributes to the smooth and creamy texture of caramel confections.

Rice Krispies Treats: This no-bake dessert is made by melting marshmallows and butter together, then adding rice cereal. Milk can be included for extra creaminess and flavor.

Fruit Yogurt Parfaits: Yogurt, often made from milk, is used in layered desserts like yogurt parfaits, where it's combined with fruits, granola, and honey for a sweet and healthy treat.

Baklava: In Middle Eastern cuisine, baklava is a sweet pastry made with layers of phyllo dough, nuts, and a sweet syrup that often includes milk or cream.

CHAPTER ELEVEN

The Future of Dairy

As we stand at the threshold of a new era, the dairy industry is poised to embrace innovation, sustainability, and adaptability like never before. This chapter explores the exciting possibilities and challenges that lie ahead for the future of dairy.

Innovation in Dairy Products

The chapter will begin by discussing the innovative trends in dairy products. Readers will learn about cutting-edge dairy products, including plant-based alternatives, functional foods, and dairy innovations that cater to evolving consumer preferences.

Innovation in the dairy industry has led to the development of a wide range of dairy products that cater to evolving consumer preferences and changing dietary needs. These innovations include:

Plant-Based Dairy Alternatives: The rise of dairy alternatives, such as almond milk, soy milk, and oat milk, reflects the growing demand for plant-based options. These products are often fortified to provide nutrients like calcium and vitamin D.

Greek Yogurt: Greek yogurt is strained to remove excess whey, resulting in a thicker and creamier product with higher protein content. It has gained popularity for its taste and nutritional profile.

Lactose-Free and Reduced-Lactose Products: Lactose-free dairy products are designed for individuals with lactose intolerance. They are treated with enzymes to break down lactose. Additionally, there are reduced-lactose options for those with mild lactose sensitivity.

Probiotic Yogurts: Yogurts with added probiotics, such as Lactobacillus and Bifidobacterium strains, promote gut health and the growth of beneficial bacteria.

High-Protein Dairy Products: Dairy companies have introduced high-protein milk, yogurt, and cheese to meet the demands of consumers looking to increase their protein intake.

Flavored Milk: Flavored milk, including chocolate, strawberry, and vanilla, continues to be a favorite among consumers, especially children. These products are sweetened and often fortified with vitamins and minerals.

Dairy Snacks: Individual-sized dairy snacks, such as yogurt cups, cheese sticks, and cottage cheese cups, provide convenient, on-the-go options for busy consumers.

Dairy-Based Desserts: Innovations in dairy desserts include artisanal ice creams, gourmet yogurts, and premium custards. These products often feature unique flavors and high-quality ingredients.

Organic and Grass-Fed Dairy: Organic and grass-fed dairy products are produced using more sustainable and ethical farming practices, which appeal to consumers looking for environmentally friendly and humane options.

A2 Milk: A2 milk is marketed as a type of milk that contains only A2 beta-casein proteins, which some individuals find easier to digest than A1 beta-casein proteins found in regular milk.

Dairy-Free Cheese: Dairy-free cheese options, made from ingredients like nuts or soy, cater to vegans and those with dairy allergies. Some of these products closely mimic the taste and texture of traditional cheese.

Functional Dairy Products: Functional dairy products are enhanced with specific nutrients or bioactive compounds, such as omega-3 fatty acids, phytosterols, and added vitamins, to address specific health needs.

Single-Origin and Artisanal Dairy Products: Specialty dairy products produced by small-scale and artisanal dairies are sought after for their unique flavors and high quality.

Reduced-Fat and Low-Sugar Dairy: Health-conscious consumers are looking for dairy products with reduced fat and sugar content while still maintaining good taste and texture.

Packaging Innovations: Eco-friendly and convenient packaging options, such as portion-controlled containers and recyclable materials, are becoming increasingly popular.

Sustainability in Dairy Farming

Sustainability is a central theme for the future of dairy farming. Readers will explore the initiatives, practices, and technologies aimed at reducing the environmental footprint of dairy production, from cow comfort and waste reduction to carbon-neutral dairy farms.

Sustainability in dairy farming is a critical consideration as the industry seeks to balance the economic, environmental, and social aspects of its operations. Here are some of the key sustainability practices and initiatives in dairy farming:

Efficient Resource Management: Dairy farms are increasingly adopting technologies and practices to improve resource efficiency. This includes optimizing feed usage, water management, and energy efficiency to reduce waste and environmental impact.

Reduced Greenhouse Gas Emissions: Dairy farms are exploring ways to mitigate their carbon footprint. This includes capturing and using methane emissions for energy, improving manure management to reduce methane, and adopting cleaner energy sources.

Animal Welfare: Ensuring the well-being of dairy cows is a sustainability priority. Farms are implementing better animal husbandry practices, providing comfortable living conditions, and offering access to open spaces to promote the physical and emotional health of the animals.

Biodiversity Conservation: Dairy farms are increasingly recognizing the importance of preserving and enhancing biodiversity on their lands. This can include creating natural habitats for wildlife, maintaining water quality, and protecting local ecosystems.

Water Management: Efficient water use and water quality protection are crucial for sustainable dairy farming. Farms are implementing measures to reduce water usage, prevent pollution, and manage runoff effectively.

Sustainable Feed Sourcing: Dairy farmers are working to source feed sustainably. This can involve using locally produced feed, implementing practices that reduce deforestation and habitat destruction, and adopting organic or non-GMO feed options.

Organic and Grass-Fed Farming: Organic dairy farming and grass-fed practices are growing in popularity due to their alignment with sustainability principles. These methods prioritize natural feed, reduced chemical use, and more humane animal treatment.

Waste Management: Managing and utilizing waste products efficiently is a sustainability practice. Dairy farms are exploring options like turning manure into fertilizer, composting, or converting waste into biogas for energy production.

Education and Training: Sustainable practices require education and training for dairy farmers. They need to stay updated on the latest sustainable technologies and techniques to implement them effectively.

Certification Programs: Many dairy farms participate in certification programs that verify their adherence to specific sustainability criteria, such as those related to organic farming, animal welfare, or environmental conservation.

Local and Community Engagement: Engaging with local communities and consumers can foster sustainability. It can involve supporting local economies, creating positive relationships with neighbors, and addressing community concerns.

Data and Technology: The use of data and technology, such as precision agriculture and data analytics, enables dairy farms to make informed decisions, optimize their operations, and reduce resource use.

Government Incentives and Regulations: Government programs and regulations can incentivize and enforce sustainable practices in the dairy industry. This can include financial incentives for adopting environmentally friendly practices and regulations on waste management and emissions.

The Rise of Dairy Tech

Readers will gain insight into the digital and technological advancements in dairy farming. This section will discuss how data analytics, robotics, and automation are transforming dairy operations, from milking to herd management.

The rise of dairy technology, also known as "dairy tech," has transformed the dairy industry by introducing innovative solutions that improve efficiency, animal welfare, and sustainability. Here are some key areas in which dairy technology has made a significant impact:

Precision Agriculture: Dairy tech utilizes precision agriculture techniques to optimize various aspects of dairy farming, such as feed management, herd health monitoring, and manure management. This technology includes sensors, data analytics, and automation to make data-driven decisions and reduce resource waste.

Milk Quality and Safety: Dairy tech has improved milk quality and safety by incorporating automated milking machines, electronic udder health monitors, and milk testing equipment. These technologies help ensure the production of high-quality, safe dairy products.

Robotic Milking Systems: Robotic milking systems have revolutionized the milking process by allowing cows to be milked on their own schedule. These systems use automated robotic arms to clean, milk, and monitor the health of cows, reducing labor requirements and improving animal welfare.

Herd Health Monitoring: Dairy tech includes wearable devices and sensors that continuously monitor the health and behavior of dairy cows. These devices can detect early signs of illness, optimize breeding schedules, and improve overall herd management.

Sustainable Farming Practices: Dairy technology supports sustainable farming practices through the use of precision equipment and data analytics to reduce water and energy consumption, minimize waste, and lower greenhouse gas emissions.

Cow Comfort and Welfare: Innovations in dairy tech include cow monitoring systems that track factors like heat stress, comfort, and behavior. This information helps farmers create better living conditions for their cows, leading to improved welfare and increased milk production.

Automated Feeding Systems: Automated feeding systems can precisely mix and distribute feed to cows, ensuring they receive the right nutrition. These systems can also reduce feed waste and labor costs.

Data Analytics and Farm Management Software: Dairy tech relies on data analytics and farm management software to collect and analyze data from various farm operations. Farmers can make data-driven decisions to optimize their operations, increase efficiency, and improve productivity.

Environmental Monitoring: Technology is used to monitor and manage environmental factors on dairy farms, such as water quality, soil health, and air quality. These insights enable farmers to reduce their environmental impact and comply with regulations.

Online Marketplaces and Supply Chain Management: Digital platforms and mobile apps connect dairy farmers with buyers, suppliers, and consumers, streamlining the supply chain and ensuring efficient distribution of dairy products.

Consumer Engagement: Dairy tech has expanded to engage consumers through traceability and transparency initiatives. Consumers can use apps and websites to learn about the source of their dairy products and the farming practices behind them.

Smart Equipment and Machinery: Modern dairy farms utilize smart equipment and machinery, including self-propelled forage harvesters, manure spreaders, and feeding robots, to increase efficiency and reduce labor costs.

The rise of dairy tech has had a profound impact on the dairy industry, enhancing efficiency, sustainability, and animal welfare. These innovations continue to evolve as technology advances, making dairy farming more efficient, profitable, and environmentally friendly.

Plant-Based Dairy Alternatives

The chapter will delve into the growing market for plant-based dairy alternatives. Readers will understand the reasons behind the rise of plant-based milk, cheese, and yogurt and the role of these alternatives in addressing consumer concerns.

Plant-based dairy alternatives have gained popularity in recent years as consumers seek dairy-free options for various reasons, including lactose intolerance, dietary preferences, and environmental concerns. These alternatives are made from a variety of plant sources and aim to mimic the taste and texture of traditional dairy products. Here are some common plant-based dairy alternatives:

Soy Milk: Soy milk is one of the most popular and widely available plant-based milk alternatives. It is made from whole soybeans and is known for its high protein content. Soy milk can be used in a similar way to cow's milk in cooking, baking, and beverages.

Almond Milk: Almond milk is made from ground almonds and water. It has a mild, slightly nutty flavor and is often lower in calories than cow's milk. Almond milk is commonly used in cereals, coffee, and smoothies.

Oat Milk: Oat milk is made from whole oats blended with water. It has a creamy texture and a mild, slightly sweet flavor. Oat milk is a versatile option for coffee, baking, and making creamy sauces.

Coconut Milk: Coconut milk is derived from the flesh of coconuts and is often used in both sweet and savory dishes. It has a rich, tropical flavor and is available in canned or carton forms. Coconut milk can add a creamy consistency to curries, soups, and desserts.

Rice Milk: Rice milk is made from milled rice and water. It has a neutral taste and is a good option for those with nut or soy allergies. Rice milk is commonly used in cereals and baking.

Cashew Milk: Cashew milk is created by blending cashews with water. It has a creamy texture and a mild, nutty flavor. Cashew milk works well in smoothies, coffee, and creamy pasta dishes.

Hemp Milk: Hemp milk is made from hemp seeds and water. It has a nutty and earthy flavor and is a good source of omega-3 fatty acids. Hemp milk is used in various recipes, including smoothies and cereals.

Pea Milk: Pea milk is a relatively new addition to the plant-based milk market. It is made from yellow peas and offers a high protein content. Pea milk can be used as a milk substitute in many applications.

Flax Milk: Flax milk is produced by blending flaxseeds and water. It has a slightly nutty taste and is rich in omega-3 fatty acids. Flax milk can be used in breakfast cereals and as a milk alternative in recipes.

Macadamia Milk: Macadamia milk is made from macadamia nuts and water. It has a creamy texture and a mild, buttery flavor. Macadamia milk is a suitable choice for coffee, baking, and cooking.

These plant-based dairy alternatives are available in various flavors, including original, unsweetened, vanilla, and chocolate. They can be used as substitutes for dairy milk in a wide range of recipes, making them accessible options for those who follow vegetarian, vegan, or lactose-free diets. Additionally, plant-based dairy alternatives contribute to reducing the environmental impact associated with traditional dairy farming.

The Evolution of Dairy Regulations

The future of dairy includes evolving regulations and standards. Readers will learn about the changes in labeling, health claims, and sustainability certifications that are shaping the dairy industry.

The evolution of dairy regulations has been driven by a combination of factors, including public health concerns, technological advancements, changing industry practices, and consumer demands. These regulations aim to ensure the safety, quality, and integrity of dairy products while protecting the interests of both consumers and dairy producers. Here's an overview of the key stages in the evolution of dairy regulations:

Early Informal Regulations (Pre-20th Century): In the early days of dairy farming, regulations were informal and often community-based. Milk quality was determined by local customs and traditions, and dairy producers were expected to adhere to certain standards of cleanliness and integrity. These standards were not standardized or enforced by any central authority.

Pasteurization and the Rise of Food Safety (Late 19th Century): The invention of pasteurization by Louis Pasteur in the late 19th century marked a significant development in dairy safety. Pasteurization, a process of heating milk to kill harmful pathogens, became a standard practice to improve the safety of dairy products.

The Establishment of the FDA (1906): The U.S. Food and Drug Administration (FDA) was established in 1906 with the passage of the Pure Food and Drug Act. This marked a significant step in regulating food safety, including dairy products, at the federal level.

National Dairy Regulation (Early to Mid-20th Century): In the early to mid-20th century, the federal government in the United States began to establish regulations related to dairy products. This included standards for milk composition, pasteurization, and labeling.

Milk Marketing Orders (1930s and 1940s): Milk marketing orders, overseen by the U.S. Department of Agriculture (USDA), were introduced to regulate the marketing and pricing of milk and dairy products. These orders aimed to stabilize dairy prices and ensure a fair return for dairy producers.

Grade A Pasteurized Milk Ordinance (PMO) (1950s): The Grade A Pasteurized Milk Ordinance (PMO) was developed to standardize the pasteurization and processing of milk at the state level in the United States. It includes regulations related to milk quality, equipment standards, and inspections.

HACCP and Modern Food Safety Practices (Late 20th Century): In the late 20th century, Hazard Analysis and Critical Control Points (HACCP) became a prominent system for ensuring food safety, including in the dairy industry. HACCP identifies and controls potential hazards in food production.

International Harmonization (Late 20th Century): The Codex Alimentarius, a global standard-setting body for food safety and quality, began to establish international dairy product standards to facilitate international trade and harmonize regulations.

Modern Dairy Labeling and Ingredient Regulations: In recent years, regulations related to dairy labeling have evolved to address issues such as the use of dairy-related terms on plant-based products. Regulators have sought to clarify labeling rules and prevent consumer confusion.

Sustainable Practices and Environmental Regulations: There is an increasing emphasis on sustainability and environmental concerns in dairy regulations. This includes regulations related to water use, waste management, and greenhouse gas emissions.

Genetic Engineering and Biotechnology: The use of biotechnology in dairy, such as the development of genetically modified organisms (GMOs) for animal feed or recombinant bovine somatotropin (rBST) for increased milk production, has led to regulations and labeling requirements.

Embracing the Future of Dairy

As the chapter wraps up, readers will recognize that the future of dairy is one of adaptation, innovation, and sustainability. They will appreciate the role of dairy in providing nourishment, supporting communities, and contributing to the global food landscape.

"Embracing the Future of Dairy" signifies the dairy industry's commitment to meeting the challenges and opportunities of a rapidly changing world. The future of dairy is characterized by several key trends and developments, each of which presents both challenges and chances for innovation and growth. Here are some of the critical aspects of embracing the future of dairy:

Sustainability: As environmental concerns become more prominent, the dairy industry is embracing sustainable practices. This includes reducing greenhouse gas emissions, minimizing water usage, and implementing eco-friendly technologies.

Technological Advancements: The dairy sector is rapidly adopting advanced technologies such as precision agriculture, data analytics, and automation. These innovations enhance efficiency, animal welfare, and product quality.

Diversification of Dairy Products: The future of dairy involves a broader range of product offerings to meet changing consumer preferences. This includes plant-based dairy alternatives, lactose-free options, and functional dairy products with added health benefits.

Globalization and Trade: The dairy industry is increasingly global, with the potential for expanded trade in dairy products. This presents opportunities to reach new markets but also requires adherence to international regulations and quality standards.

Transparency and Traceability: Consumers are demanding more transparency in the food supply chain. Dairy producers are embracing technologies like blockchain to provide consumers with detailed information about the source and journey of dairy products.

Health and Wellness: Dairy is evolving to meet the growing demand for healthier options. This includes reduced-fat and reduced-sugar products, as well as dairy items with functional ingredients designed to promote well-being.

Alternative Production Methods: Some dairy products are being created through innovative methods, such as cellular agriculture and fermentation. These approaches offer more sustainable and resource-efficient ways of producing dairy.

Consumer Engagement: Dairy producers are actively engaging with consumers through social media, marketing, and educational campaigns to better understand and address consumer preferences.

Regulatory Compliance: The dairy industry is adapting to evolving regulatory requirements, including those related to labeling, food safety, and environmental practices.

Collaboration and Research: Collaboration between the dairy industry, research institutions, and government agencies is essential to address current and future challenges. Research into new technologies, animal health, and nutrition is key to continued progress.

Resilience and Adaptation: Dairy producers are embracing strategies to enhance resilience in the face of climate change, economic fluctuations, and global health crises, such as the COVID-19 pandemic.

Quality Assurance: Maintaining the high quality and safety of dairy products remains a top priority. Producers are investing in quality control measures and certifications to meet consumer expectations.

In summary, "Embracing the Future of Dairy" means proactively addressing the challenges and opportunities presented by evolving consumer preferences, technology, sustainability concerns, and globalization. It involves a commitment to responsible practices, innovation, and the continued production of high-quality dairy products that meet the needs of consumers while respecting the planet's resources.

Epilogue

In this final chapter of "The Milky Way: Exploring the World of Dairy," we reflect on the vast and rich landscape of the dairy industry, tracing the journey of milk from the cow to your glass, and exploring the world of dairy in all its forms. We've embarked on a journey that has taken us through the pastures and parlor, uncovered the history of dairy farming, delved into the diverse breeds of dairy cows, and traced the transformation of raw milk into refined dairy products.

We've marveled at the nutrient powerhouse that is milk, with its ability to support bone health, cardiovascular wellness, weight management, and more. We've celebrated the dairy world's masterpiece, cheese, from its mysterious origins to its diverse and complex flavors. We've savored the richness of butter and cream, exploring their pivotal roles in the culinary arts.

We've immersed ourselves in the world of yogurt and fermented delights, uncovering their cultural significance and their impact on gut health. We've scrutinized the intricate connection between dairy and human health, from bone and dental health to heart health and immune support. We've appreciated the enduring presence of milk in our culinary endeavors, from baking to sauces, soups, desserts, and beyond.

And we’ve peered into the future of dairy, witnessing the exciting possibilities and challenges that lie ahead. The dairy industry is evolving, embracing innovation, sustainability, and adaptability, and we’ve explored the growing interest in plant-based dairy alternatives, technological advancements in dairy farming, and the quest for sustainability and health.

As our journey through "The Milky Way" comes to a close, we’re left with a profound understanding of the dairy industry’s significance in our lives, our health, and our culinary traditions. Dairy is not merely a collection of products but a reflection of our history, our culture, and our ever-changing world.

We invite you to continue your exploration of the world of dairy, whether it’s by savoring your favorite cheese, experimenting with dairy-inspired recipes, or delving deeper into the science and culture of dairy. The Milky Way is an ever-expanding universe of discovery, and we hope you’ll continue to explore it with enthusiasm and appreciation.

Thank you for joining us on this journey through "The Milky Way," and may your appreciation for the world of dairy continue to grow, enriching your culinary experiences and your understanding of the world of agriculture and nutrition.

.....***.....

www.ingramcontent.com/pod-product-compliance
Lightning Source LLC
Chambersburg PA
CBHW050759260726
48660CB00004B/1157
* 9 7 9 8 8 6 5 8 1 1 8 3 1 *